GO
TO
BED

The Clinician's Handbook
for Understanding SLEEP

Andrew Koppejan, PT

Published by Clinical Marketing Inc.

Edmonton, Alberta, Canada

ISBN: 978-0-9959954-1-3

TABLE OF CONTENTS

WHY THIS BOOK?
By the Author

With nearly one-third of our lives spent sleeping, it's something that we can often take for granted.

Until our sleep becomes disrupted.

Whether through personal stress, injury, or the myriad of other instigating factors, our sleep can become disturbed and its impacts can be far reaching. Our ability to think clearly, treat others with care, or function becomes impaired.

As health care providers, we work with patients who have disrupted sleep. Yet often we avoid conversations about sleep health. Addressing sleep with our patients can provide an opportunity to more fully treat the whole person.

By helping our patients with their sleep, we can support their physical recovery and return to greater levels of function. Healthy sleep equals a healthy body.

We are all too aware of the increasing prevalence of chronic or persistent pain in our society and in our patient populations. And whether a triggering or resulting factor, sleep is impacted.

It's an active process of recovery for the body and impaired sleep can impact healthy functioning, healthy beliefs and cognitions and recovery of acute or chronic injuries.

Prior to my research, I would have conversations with patients about their sleep issues and would quickly exhaust my education—limited to commonly known sleep hygiene rules. I was frustrated with my lack of knowledge in this important area and frustrated with my inability to engage in more transformative conversations with my patients.

When researching this topic online, you'll find a plethora of sleep information tidbits, but nothing that helps identify and summarize the specifics used to help health care clinicians with their patients.

The purpose of this book is to provide a concise, practical handbook for health care providers to assist their patients with sleep. I reviewed over 170 academic journal articles along with a multitude of sleep science textbooks and popular sleep help books. From this research, I pulled out the most important information related to sleep health and wellness.

I hope you find this book, and the associated resources, a valuable clinical resource that will improve your care of patients with sleep disturbance.

To better sleep,

Andrew Koppejan, PT

AUTHOR
Andrew Koppejan, PT

Nearly one-third of our lives are spent sleeping, so when our sleep is disrupted it has immediate effects on our ability to think, act and reason clearly.

Andrew Koppejan, a registered physiotherapist and founder of ignitephysio, an online learning community, has spent the better part of his medical professional life seeking to improve connection and collaboration between medical professionals for the benefit of patients. Certified in GunnIMS, Koppejan regularly works with chronic pain patients and has seen the powerful relationship between sleep and pain.

Through over 170 academic articles, textbooks and popular sleep help books, Koppejan has sought answers to the enigmatic relationship between sleep and health, knowing already that "healthy sleep equals a healthy body," but missing the "why."

Health care providers are in a unique position to deliver the keys to great sleep health and this book is the perfect concise, practical handbook to do just that.

Research Contributors

A special thank you to physiotherapists Meaghan Clarke and Nani Woollings for their work to support the research efforts with this project.

COMMON SLEEP TERMS

Understand the terminology and acronyms used in the evaluation and treatment of sleep.

There are a number of commonly used terms in sleep research and sleep outcome measures. This list will be helpful in your own reading about sleep health as well as in your conversations with patients and other healthcare providers.

COMMON SLEEP DEFINITIONS

Sleep Architecture

Refers to the general structural organization of normal sleep. This includes the alternating, cyclical states of sleep known as REM and NREM sleep which are defined by EEG readings.[1]

Short Wave Sleep

Alpha or short wave sleep is characterized by low amplitude, high frequency wave patterns.

Slow Wave Sleep (SWS)

Delta wave sleep or deep wave sleep is characterized by high amplitude, slow frequency wave patterns and occurs during the third stage of NREM sleep known as N3.

Sleep Fragmentation

This refers to interruption of sleep throughout the night. There is a hierarchy of fragmentation:

Micro-arousals: Abrupt shift in alpha, theta, and/or delta EEG waves that last between 3 to 10 seconds

Awakenings: Responses that last more than 10 seconds

Wakefulness: return of full arousal

Sleep Stage Shift: when an individual moves from a deeper to a lighter sleep state e.g. slow wave sleep (N3) to Stage 1 or 2 (N1 or N2).[2]

Sleep Inertia

Sleep inertia explains the grogginess that we feel upon waking. Sleep inertia is greater when we attempt to wake outside of our circadian rhythm or during deep sleep.[3]

COMMON SLEEP DIARY TERMS

The following sleep terms are frequently seen in sleep research, used in sleep diaries (e.g. Consensus Sleep Diary), sleep outcome measures and objective sleep testing:

Total Sleep Time (TST)

This is the average total nighttime sleep and is typically recorded in a sleep diary. It is measured in minutes.

Time in Bed (TIB)

This is the total amount of time spent in bed from when the lights go out to when one gets out of bed.

Total Wake Time (TWT)

This accounts for all time awake while in bed including time to fall asleep, awake time during the night, as well as awake time prior to getting out of bed in the morning.

Wake After Sleep Onset (WASO)

This is the amount of time spent awake during the night after initially falling asleep. It is measured in minutes.

Sleep Efficiency (SE%)

This is the total sleep time (TST) divided by average time spent in bed (TIB). The sleep efficiency formula can be expressed as (100 x [TST/ TIB]). It is recorded as a percentage.

Sleep Onset Latency (SOL)

The amount of time it takes to transition from wakefulness to sleep.

CHAPTER 1

WHEN SLEEP GOES WRONG

Understand the prevalence of disrupted sleep and the key health impacts of poor sleep.

COVERED IN THIS CHAPTER:
Understanding Disrupted Sleep
Effects of Sleep Deprivation
Health Impacts of Disrupted Sleep

UNDERSTANDING DISRUPTED SLEEP

Disrupted sleep is a significant problem in our society and can affect people across the lifespan.

The Problem

Poor sleep is a growing problem and one that affects a large number of people. In the United States, an estimated 50-70 million adults suffer from a sleep or wakefulness disorder. Almost 20% of all serious car accidents, independent of alcohol, are a result of driver sleepiness.[1] It has been reported that one third of the adult population is affected by insomnia occasionally and between 9-12% on a chronic basis.[4]

There are a significant number of Americans who suffer from other sleep disorders:

- 3 to 4 million suffer from moderate to severe obstructive sleep apnea
- 15 million (5% of the general population) suffer from restless leg syndrome and periodic limb movement disorders[1]

In a survey of 2,000 Canadians, nearly 20% said they were dissatisfied with their sleep, and 40% had more than one symptom of insomnia including trouble falling or staying asleep, or early morning awakening and 14% had met all the criteria for insomnia.[5]

Disturbed sleep can be defined when one or more of these problems is present:

- Insomnia
- Abnormal movements, and sensations or behaviors during sleep or during nocturnal waking
- Excessive sleepiness during the day[6]

Understanding the Impact

We don't have to look far at the impact of disrupted sleep in society. Just look at colossal tragedies including the disasters of Chernobyl and the Exxon Valdez, among others. Each of these had fatigue-related performance errors. Although disrupted sleep doesn't always show up in significant ways, disrupted sleep, including chronic insomnia, have a significant impact on our economies and society as a whole.

In comparison to healthy sleepers, those with sleep loss have been found to experience greater health care needs such as emergency and health care visits, as well as increased prescription medications.[7] They also experience an increased likelihood of injury. In fact, it is estimated that 110,000 sleep related injuries and 5,000 fatalities result from car accidents involving commercial trucks.[1]

There are a number of indirect costs associated with insomnia which include increased missed work days and loss of productivity. While it has been estimated that direct costs associated with insomnia in the USA are between $2 to 16 billion per year, indirect costs soar all the way to $75-100 billion per year.[7]

Understanding Those Affected

It is important to understand those who are more likely to be affected by, and are at risk for, disturbed sleep. Here is a summary of key demographic segments who are at a greater risk of disrupted sleep including insomnia:

> **Age:** Insomnia increases with age. The odds of experiencing chronic insomnia increases 1.1 fold for every decade of life and there is almost a doubling of insomnia in those greater than 75 years of age.[8] In fact, the elderly have a 1.5x higher rate of difficulty falling asleep and elderly women use more hypnotics to improve their sleep.[9]

Female: Women are more likely to suffer from insomnia. Insomnia rates are double that of men across the lifespan and studies show a consistent increased risk ratio for women (range of 1.32 to 1.64).[8]

Lower Socioeconomic Class: Both lower socioeconomic class and education levels affect sleep quality.[8]

Older adults are at risk for disrupted sleep including insomnia. As we age, sleep quality is impacted by inactivity, decreased light exposure, decreased arousal threshold, elevated autonomic activity and changes to circadian rhythms.[10]

However, disrupted sleep isn't partial to adults. Children can also suffer from sleep problems. In fact, approximately 40-45% of children will experience sleep disorders during infancy and adolescence. Insomnia has been found to occur in 20% of children on a regular basis.[11]

EFFECTS OF SLEEP DEPRIVATION

Both total and partial sleep deprivation have significant effects on physical and psychological well-being.

Sleep Deficiency

Even though it is easy to dismiss poor sleep as a reality of the modern life, the impacts on our health are many. By understanding the impacts of poor sleep caused by insomnia, we can help communicate the importance of sleep and the value of addressing sleep issues to enhance recovery and improve overall health.

Sleep deficiency can be defined as insufficient quantity or inadequate quality of sleep obtained relative to that needed for optimal health, performance and well-being.[12]

Fatigue following 20-25 hours of awake time impairs performing tasks to the same level of alcohol intoxication at a 0.10% blood level concentration (legally drunk in many jurisdictions).[13]

Effects of Total Sleep Deprivation

Total sleep deprivation highlights the significant impacts on psychological and physiological function. These have been described in the literature[13,14,15]:

Psychological Effects:

- Impaired attention and loss of concentration
- Longer reaction time
- Slowed reasoning
- Distractedness
- Increased stress
- Impaired creative thinking
- Deterioration of short-term memory and consolidation of long-term memory
- Irritability and mood disturbance
- Loss of motivation
- Fear, frustration and/or anger of being unable to sleep

Physical Effects:

- Physical weariness, fatigue and tiredness
- Muscle aches, including headaches and neck pain, due to the lack of muscle motor inhibition normally observed during sleep
- Exacerbation of tremors, intensifying the longer the reduction in sleep lasts
- Decreased postural control and balance
- Reduced anaerobic power
- Double vision or tunnel vision
- Greater number of visual errors or hallucinations
- Difficulty verbalizing and experiencing thoughts and concepts
- Slowed speech, stammering, monotone expression
- Increased use of word repetitions and clichés

Although total sleep deprivation studies help to more clearly identify the physiological effects, partial and acute sleep restriction can help to give us a better sense of the impacts associated with everyday life. Not only do total sleep deprivation studies show significant changes to various homeostatic health systems, but partial sleep deprivation studies, which more closely mimic real life, also show remarkable changes within the body.

The impacts of poor sleep are many. Once you begin to discover the impact of poor sleep on general health, you will begin to appreciate the need for a higher level of importance to be placed on sleep health.

HEALTH IMPACTS OF DISRUPTED SLEEP

Chronic sleep deprivation can lead to increased obesity and diabetes risk, decreased immunity and increased inflammation.

Impacts on General Health

There are a number of general health implications resulting from poor sleep which impact interconnected areas of weight gain, glucose regulation, diabetes and hypertension. Unfortunately, the more chronic sleep deprivation becomes, the greater the risk for developing a variety of co-morbidities (hypertension, dyslipidemia, diabetes, obesity) as well as a reduced ability to tolerate stressful stimuli.[14,16,17]

The following table highlights the increased prevalence of various medical disorders reported by those with insomnia versus those without insomnia[8]:

Medical Problem	Prevalence in those with Insomnia	Prevalence in those without insomnia
Heart disease	22%	9%
Cancer	9%	4%
Hypertension	43%	19%
Neurologic Disease	7%	1%
Diabetes	13%	5%
Chronic Pain	50%	18%

Note: Adapted from Lichstein et al. (Numbers have been rounded)

As you can see from this table, the prevalence of medical problems is increased significantly in those with insomnia.

Altered sleep also impacts mortality. In one study, the risk of death increases by 12% for those that get less than 7 hours of sleep.[12]

Influence on Obesity And Diabetes

The rising epidemic of obesity and diabetes in North America is alarming. As movement experts, the significant effects on mobility and function are a significant cause for concern. Research has shown that there is relationship between weight gain, obesity and poor sleep.[14, 16] Authors Buxton et al, argue that in addition to the pillars of exercise and diet, sleep should be included as a primary pillar of health.

It appears that even when confounding variables such as obesity and overweight are removed, sleep is independently related to diabetes risk. In a pooled analyses of over 100,000 adults, sleeping less than 6 hours per night had a RR (risk ratio) of 1.28 in predicting T2DM and over sleeping (>8-9 hours) resulted in a RR of 1.48. Difficulty falling asleep and staying asleep also had a strong relationship with diabetes risk (RR 1.48, RR 1.84).[12]

The increase in weight gain associated with decreased sleep appears to have a few different connections:

- Studies have shown that hormones such as ghrelin (appetite stimulant) increase and appetite suppressing hormones (leptin) decrease with reduced sleep.

- There is an altered brain response to food. Specifically, there is an increased desirability for food through activating the central reward systems and a decrease in self-control.

- Energy expenditure is altered, including the resting metabolic rate (RMR).[12]

In one particular controlled study, participants who were put on a sleep restricted program (4 hours per night) showed a 15% increase in food intake and a 39% increase in fat consumption.

Glucose regulation also appears to be affected by partial sleep deprivation. A number of studies show glucose dysregulation and decreased insulin sensitivity as a result of impaired sleep. Important to glucose regulation is the hormone cortisol. Whether with total or partial sleep deprivation, cortisol has been shown to increase (45% vs 37%) the following day altering 24- hour cortisol profiles.[12]

Impacts on Immune Function

When it comes to the effect that sleep deprivation has on our immunity, there is still a lot to learn. Although the majority of studies investigating this relationship have been done on rats, preliminary findings suggest that sleep is an important key in immunity.[18]

What we know so far is that physical restoration occurs during deep or slow wave sleep (SWS).[14] When sleep loss reduces time spent here, our body's ability to rejuvenate is inhibited. From a micro level, sleep deprivation has a negative effect on cell immunity and cytokine function. Without adequate sleep, there is a reduction in the function of peripheral blood lymphocytes and natural killer cells, as well as an increase in inflammatory markers such as interleukin and tumor necrosis factor.[14,16,18] With such physiological changes, there comes an increased susceptibility to infections, a poor ability to fight infections and a greater incidence of sepsis.[18]

Impact on Inflammation

As we know, inflammation is a non-specific immune response that is usually activated when the body experiences injury or infection. It can sometimes be activated with disease and some genetic predispositions.[19]

Insomnia and sleep deprivation can result in increases in a variety of inflammatory processes—pro-inflammatory effects—which can cause negative effects on health.[19] Pro-inflammatory responses involve increased cytokine secretion ex: IL-1, tumor necrosis factor (TNF) and IL-6, and increased circulating monocytes, NK cells, and CRP.[20,21,22]

As well, studies are showing that the relationship of inflammation and sleep deprivation may be bidirectional: sleep dysfunction can cause inflammation, and the inflammatory response can alter sleep quality and quantity.[19]

Key Take-Aways

- A significant number of people suffer from disrupted sleep.

- Sleep deprivation has wide ranging effects on human functioning and performance.

- Insomnia is associated with a number of medical problems and contributes to increased risk of obesity, hypertension and diabetes.

- Immune function can become impaired with sleep deprivation and sleep deprivation contributes to increased inflammation in the body.

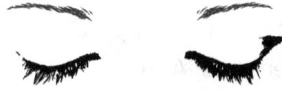

CHAPTER 2

UNDERSTANDING INSOMNIA AND OTHER SLEEP DISORDERS

Increase your confidence in understanding the condition of insomnia and other possible causes of poor sleep.

COVERED IN THIS CHAPTER:
Defining Insomnia
Additional Sleep Disorders
Depression & Sleep

DEFINING INSOMNIA

Insomnia, the difficulty of sleeping, is the most common sleep disorder. According to the National Sleep Foundation, which Peter Hauri references in his book *The Sleep Disorders*, insomnia affects as many as 30 million Americans. A 2005 survey conveys that one-third of respondents experienced at least one symptom of insomnia every night or almost every night.[23] Although approximately 30% of adults will report experiencing insomnia symptoms, only about 6-10% meet insomnia disorder criteria.[24]

Defining insomnia has been a challenge in the medical community. It can be a symptom of another disorder while also being its own disorder and insomnia symptoms can morph into an insomnia disorder. In addition, insomnia is a heterogeneous condition with varying causes, durations and types.[8]

Part of the challenge in defining insomnia is that the diagnosis of insomnia is based on patient report. Interestingly, objective sleep analysis (e.g. polysomnography or actigraphy) isn't very sensitive in distinguishing those with and without insomnia, and patient self-report often doesn't correlate strongly to objective sleep data.[25] This difference highlights that those with insomnia have altered perception of their sleep.

There are a number of different classification systems that define insomnia including:

- **DSM:** from the American Psychiatric Association (current version: DSM-V)

- **ICSD:** from the American Academy of Sleep Medicine (current version: ICSD-2)

- **ICD:** from the World Health Organization (current version: ICD-10)

One of the challenges with defining insomnia is that definitions vary across these different classification systems. Lichstein et al[26] reviewed the different definitions and highlighted the lack of consistency between these classification systems. The latest versions are narrowing the gap between the definition of insomnia.

In its essence, insomnia can be defined as a person expressing difficulty falling asleep or staying asleep. Difficulties staying asleep could include difficulties returning to sleep after awakening or waking earlier than desired with the inability to fall back asleep. Those with insomnia differ from healthy sleepers in that they typically take more than 30 minutes to fall asleep and/or will be awake for more than 30 minutes during the night.[25]

Research also indicates that those with insomnia may also complain of non-restorative sleep. It's important to note that one should have adequate opportunity for sleep (as opposed to sleep deprivation). Also important is the requirement that insomnia have some impact on daytime functioning.[25]

Roth, in his article "Insomnia: Definition, Prevalence, Etiology & Consequences" defined insomnia like this:

- Difficulty falling asleep, staying asleep or non-restorative sleep
- Difficulty occurs despite sufficient opportunity and circumstance for sleep
- Associated with daytime impairment
- Occurs at least 3 times per week, lasting longer than at least one month[27]

A helpful way of defining insomnia is that insomnia symptoms should include one sleep symptom and one waking symptom.

Sleep symptoms may include:

- Difficulty falling asleep
- Difficulty staying asleep
- Early morning awakening
- Non-refreshing sleep

Awake symptoms can include self-reports of:

- Sleepiness
- Fatigue
- Mood disturbance (e.g. irritability)
- Cognitive difficulties
- Social impairment
- Occupational impairment (prone to errors or accidents)[8]

Traditionally, insomnia has been classified as either primary or secondary. Primary insomnia is a loss of sleep that has no identifiable cause whereas secondary insomnia is loss of sleep due to causes such as illness, drugs, and health conditions such as depression. With the new edition of the Diagnostic and Statistical Manual of Mental Disorders (DSM-V) this differentiation has been removed. However, it is helpful to understand this nuance in classification as this terminology may still come up in reading sleep health literature.

Acute And Chronic Insomnia

It's safe to say that we have all experienced acute insomnia for some reason or another; whether caused by a stressful situation like exams, jet lag, a crying baby, or pain, to name just a few!

Acute insomnia can be categorized into transient insomnia, which lasts for a few days, to short-term insomnia, which can last for several weeks.[28] It is defined as lasting less than three months with a specific triggering event.[29]

Acute insomnia can occur at times of stress, illness, altitude changes and jet lag.[28] These factors typically resolve on their own after a few days without any consequence. However, the concern is when insomnia extends past a few days into several weeks. If not properly treated, the risk of developing chronic insomnia increases.

Acute insomnia should not be trivialized since, once developed, insomnia problems tend to persist. Studies have shown that for 80% of people who experience insomnia, they will continue to experience insomnia two years later.[29] In another research study by Canadian sleep researcher Charles Morin, the author emphasizes the importance

> # Potential Causes of Acute Insomnia:
> • Bedroom environment changes
> • Background noise changes
> • Work/school demands
> • Loss of a loved one or recent divorce
> • Illness/injury causes pain
> • Caffeine usage/withdrawal
> • Work shift changes
> • Stimulant medication usage
> Source: Adapted from Bonnet et al, 2012

of not dismissing insomnia complaints. He highlights that 70% of individuals with insomnia will continue to experience insomnia one year later and 50% will continue reporting insomnia up to three years later.[30]

Sleep researchers have studied the reasons behind the transition from acute to chronic insomnia. A popular behavioral model posited by Arthur Spielman and his colleagues (as outlined by Manber & Carney) argues that chronic insomnia results from the interaction of three factors:

Trait Factors: biopsychosocial factors

Precipitating Factors: acute factors that are life stressors

Maintaining Factors: maladaptive strategies that people adopt in their attempts to improve their sleep

An individual may have a stressful event such as the loss of a family member (precipitating factor) which results in acute insomnia. This individual may then attempt to address this loss of sleep through increased napping or decreased activity (maintaining factors) resulting in decreased sleep drive ensuring that chronic insomnia results.[31]

Interestingly, the precipitating factors are no longer relevant after a certain amount of time, as conditioned sleep behaviors and persistent arousal have resulted in chronic insomnia.

ADDITIONAL SLEEP DISORDERS

There are a number of sleep disorders outside of insomnia that contribute to disrupted sleep.

There are many ways that sleep can be impacted outside of insomnia. This list is not exhaustive but will help give you an understanding of the more common sleep disorders.

Sleep Disordered Breathing (Apnea)

Obstructive sleep apnea (OSA) is the most common breathing problem in sleep, with numbers revealing that it affects between 2-26% of the general population.[32]

Obstructive sleep apnea occurs when sleep is disrupted because of partial obstruction of the airway, leading to lowered blood oxygen levels.[33] OSA is connected with loud snoring during sleep, excessive daytime sleepiness, hypertension and decreased quality of life.

OSA is more than a noisy nuisance. It has serious health implications. Those with OSA have a 20-year shorter life expectancy and those with OSA have a higher incidence of hypertension, coronary artery disease, strokes, GERD, heart failure and heart attacks.[32] Unfortunately, OSA is severely under diagnosed. In those with moderate to severe OSA, 80% of men and 93% of women were undiagnosed.

Whereas those with OSA have difficulty inhaling due to airway collapse, patients with central sleep apnea can stop breathing.

Those with central sleep apnea (CSA) have pauses in their breathing due to the absence of respiratory effort. This absence is due to a temporary loss of output from the breathing pacemaker. It is less common than obstructive sleep apnea, but the two forms of apnea can occur together. Central sleep apnea is a disorder of the central nervous system where there is disruption between the brainstem and the muscles of respiration, resulting in shortness of breath that awakens you from sleep and intermittent pauses in breathing during sleep. This can be caused by medical conditions like congestive heart failure, coronary heart disease, stroke, hypertension and opioid use.[34]

Circadian Rhythm Sleep-Wake Disorders (CRSWD)

These disorders come as a result of a disruption in the endogenous circadian rhythm and the day-night cycles become misaligned. This can lead to chronic sleep problems.[35] CRSWD can lead to cognitive, learning and behavioral/emotional impairments.[36]

Periodic Limb Movement Disorder

Periodic limb movements of sleep (PLMS) are regularly occurring movements of the lower extremity, most commonly ankle dorsiflexion and great toe flexion. PLMS is observed in around 85% of Restless Leg Syndrome (RLS) patients. RLS is a syndrome that has four defining factors:

- An urge to move the legs
- Worsens with rest
- Temporary relief with movement
- Typically occurs in the evening or at night.

In comparing RLS to neuropathy, neuropathy does not have an urge to move, nor a nocturnal preference, nor relief with movement. Whereas neuropathy tends to mainly affect the feet, RLS generally does not affect the feet.[37]

Parasomnias

Parasomnias can be classified as any undesirable behaviors that take place during sleep. This would include sleep terrors and nightmares, sleepwalking, and sleep talking, among others. Parasomnias take place during sleep transitions, and the state of wakefulness and sleep become blurred. With parasomnias, NREM and REM states can occur simultaneously or move back and forth very quickly.[38]

Narcolepsy

This is a chronic brain disorder where control over one's sleep-wake cycles is reduced. It is characterized by daytime sleepiness and sudden "sleep attacks" often accompanied by cataplexy, sleep paralysis and hypnagogic hallucinations.[39]

Narcolepsy also impacts the regulation of REM sleep. REM sleep in those with narcolepsy can occur at any time of the day and can often intrude on one's waking state resulting in atypical intermediate states (e.g. cataplexy).[39]

DEPRESSION AND SLEEP

It's important to recognize the close relationship between depression and sleep.

An Overview

When looking at disrupted sleep, I would be remiss to not discuss the relationship of poor sleep with depression.

Depression is a major healthcare problem worldwide with a reported lifetime prevalence ranging from 2% to 15% and is associated with significant disability. As well, depression has been found to impair one's health status to a greater degree than other diseases. Unfortunately, depression combined with other chronic morbidities resulted in the worst health scores for all diseases.[40]

The Relationship Between Depression And Sleep

The presence of insomnia and depression are highly interlinked. Insomnia is a diagnostic symptom of a major depressive episode according to the DSM-V.

Some interesting results were uncovered in a study looking at the relationship between depression and anxiety in 772 subjects with and without insomnia. The findings were telling as they identified the increased prevalence of psychological disturbance in those with insomnia:

- Those with insomnia were nearly 10x more likely to have clinically significant depression and 17x more likely to have clinically significant anxiety.

- The number of awakenings per night was related to increased depression scores.

- Women were more likely than men to experience insomnia and had increased levels of depression.

- 20% of people with insomnia displayed clinically significant depression and ~19% demonstrated clinically significant anxiety.[41]

It appears that insomnia can both precede or follow a depressive episode. In a study looking at this relationship, insomnia started before the depression episode for over 40% of subjects, while an equal portion of individuals started experiencing insomnia during or after their first depressive episode.[30]

As one can see, depression and insomnia are interlinked, and the relationship does not appear to be one-sided. Although it would make sense that sleep would improve once depression resolved, Manber & Carney summarize research that highlights the following:

- Poor sleep will predict future depressive episodes.

- Poor sleep is not fully resolved after depression lifts.

- Poor sleep has been shown to predict decreased response to treatment.

- Sleep challenges typically remain unresolved with anti-depressant medications and typical psychotherapy.[31]

In upcoming sections of the book, the relationship between depression, chronic pain and sleep will be discussed.

Key Take-Aways

- Defining insomnia has been a challenge and is one of the few conditions based on patient self-report.

- Those with insomnia have an altered perception of their sleep.

- Acute insomnia can transition into chronic insomnia even after precipitating events have passed.

- Always be sure to screen for other potential sleep disorders, especially sleep disordered breathing.

- Insomnia is a common symptom of depression and could be a potential cause of insomnia.

CHAPTER 3

DRUG EFFECTS ON SLEEP

There are a wide variety of prescription and recreational drugs that can impact sleep.

COVERED IN THIS CHAPTER:
Pain Medications
Mood Disorder Drugs
Cardiovascular Drugs
Antihistamines
Antiepileptic Drugs
Antiparkinson Drugs
Recreational Drugs

INTRODUCTION

Drugs can impact sleep health. Everything from anti-depressants to antihistamines, the impact of drugs on sleep is still emerging. As healthcare providers, having a basic understanding of medications that impact sleep can provide valuable insight into the influencers of sleep health in our patients.

It is important to note that questions from patients relating to their medications should be directed to their family physicians and pharmacists. For other healthcare providers, such as physiotherapists, it is important to avoid providing recommendations regarding medications as it is important to stay within one's scope of professional practice.

PAIN MEDICATIONS

NSAIDs

Unfortunately, there haven't been many studies looking at the effect of NSAIDs on sleep. In one study of healthy subjects, ASA (Aspirin) and ibuprofen disrupted total sleep by increasing awakenings and decreasing slow wave sleep.[42] These drugs decrease prostaglandin D2 which impacts melatonin synthesis and prevents body temperature lowering at night.[43] It appears that while NSAIDs are helpful to reduce arthritic pain, they don't appear to change the effects of arthritis pain on sleep architecture.[42]

Acetaminophen (Tylenol)

It appears that this drug has little effect on sleep architecture in healthy human subjects.[42]

Opioid Analgesics

Opioid analgesics have doubled in use worldwide between 2001-2003 and 2011-2013 with 94% of worldwide use coming from the USA and western and central Europe. This growth is believed to be partly due to prescribing for non-cancer pain.[44]

Opioid analgesics, which include morphine, fentanyl and codeine are commonly prescribed medications in the treatment of acute and chronic pain which is moderate to severe.[42] While these drugs have a sedative effect, they have significant impacts on sleep.

In both animal and human studies, the most significant acute effect of morphine is the significant suppression of REM sleep. This decrease in REM sleep also appears to take place throughout administration of morphine.[42] Other sleep effects from opioids include reduced sleep quality, worsened sleep latency, and decreased total sleep time.[45,46]

In an interesting study by Morasco et al, they evaluated three groups: 1) those with chronic pain taking opioids, 2) those with chronic pain, but with no opioid use and 3) those without with chronic pain. The researchers discovered:

- More sleep impairment (as measured by the PSQI) by those taking opioids for chronic pain, as compared to those not taking opioids for chronic pain

- Significant impairment in sleep latency present in those taking opioid medications

- Increased sleep apnea diagnoses in patients taking opioids for chronic pain.

In this study, nearly 25% of patients taking prescribed opioids were diagnosed with sleep apnea and the authors recommend that sleep apnea screening be done in this population.[45]

This concern with disordered breathing with opioid use is well documented. In fact, 70-85% of patients taking opioids have disordered breathing with a high number being moderate to severe.[47]

Cannabis

Cannabis, commonly known as marijuana, affects individuals differently. Although cannabis may induce relaxation and drowsiness, there are other symptoms that can take place such as mild euphoria, talkativeness, intensification of sensory experiences, difficulty concentrating and altered time perception.[48]

Cannaboids are a group of compounds found in cannabis that include cannabidiol (CBD)and D-9-tetrahydrocannabinol (THC). The psychotropic effects of cannabis are believed to come from THC.[48]

Animal studies suggest that acute use of cannaboids suppresses REM sleep, but that this effect on REM sleep dissipates rapidly with increased use.[42]

In human studies, it appears that the effects of THC differ between cannabis-naive subjects vs long-term users. There is some evidence to suggest that there may be arousing effects in those who are cannabis-naive subjects resulting in increased sleep latency (delay in falling asleep).[48]

Most significant is that human studies consistently show cannabis use decreases total REM sleep and REM density.[48] It does appear that dosing has a significant impact on wakefulness and sleep as does the ratio between CBD vs THC.[49]

In his review of cannaboids, Cairns suggests that its chronic use can modestly improve SWS, but he cautions that it is unclear whether these effects would be observed in cannabis-naive individuals or how pain could impact their effect on sleep.[42]

It is important to highlight that cannabis withdrawal can impact sleep negatively and influence strange dreams. These typically occur within 24-72 hours after ending cannabis use.[48]

MOOD DISORDER DRUGS

Antidepressants

Given that those with depression often have disrupted sleep, researchers have acknowledged the challenge with antidepressants' influence on sleep and wakefulness.

Tricyclic Antidepressants (TCAs): There are varying effects on sleep depending on the drug. Generally, these drugs increase total sleep time, decrease sleep latency, but decrease REM. Substantial REM suppression occurs with amitriptyline & doxepin.[50] Certain TCA's can worsen insomnia by increasing frequency of periodic limb movement.[43]

Monoamine oxidase inhibitors (MAOIs): These antidepressants can result in decreased REM and decreased total sleep time. Insomnia and daytime sedation are common side effects. Newer MAOIs show less adverse effects.[43]

Selective serotonin re-uptake inhibitors (SSRIs): SSRIs can result in disrupted sleep continuity and decreased REM. SSRIs can be associated with increased insomnia, sedation and PLMS.[43]

The following table summarizes common antidepressants by their class:

TCAs	MAOIs	SSRIs
Elavil (Amitriptyline)	Nardil (Phenelzine)	Celexa (Citalopram)
Asendin (Amoxapine)	Parnate (Tranylcypromine)	Lexapro (Escitalopram)
Norpramin (Desipramine)	Emsam / Zelpar (Selegiline)	Fluoxetine (Prozac)
Anafranil / Sienquan (Doxepin)		Luvox (Fluvoxamine)
Surmontil (Triminpramine)		Paxil (Paroxetine)
Tofranil (Imipramine)		Zoloft (Sertraline)

Anti-Psychotics

This would include drugs such as Zyprexa (Olanazpine), Seroquel (Quetiapine), and Geodon (Ziprasidone). These drugs have a complex pharmacological profile. Sedation is a common side effect. Patients with schizophrenia often have insomnia and circadian rhythm disorders as well as cognitive issues, so evaluating the effect of drugs on sleep is difficult.[43] It appears that newer "atypical" drugs such as olanazpine, quetiapine, risperidone and ziprasidone decrease sleep latency and improve sleep efficiency and overall sleep time.[50]

Anxiolytics (Anti-Anxiety Medications)

Benzodiazepines: Drugs in this class include Valium (Diazepam), Ativan (Lorazepam), and Xanax (Alprazolam). When used for anti-anxiety purposes, these drugs have similar pharmacological effects as the benzodiazepines used for insomnia management. The most common side effect is sedation. Performance impairment (e.g. driving) is common early in use.[43]

CARDIOVASCULAR DRUGS

Beta Blockers: CNS effects from these drugs (e.g. Acebutolol, Metoprolol, Propranolol) include tiredness, fatigue, insomnia, nightmares and vivid dreams. There is a decreased release of melatonin which may impact sleep. Propranolol, a common beta-blocker, is commonly associated with disrupted sleep. In one study, REM sleep was decreased.[43]

Statins: There are subjective reports of insomnia, however no objective measurement has shown a significant effect.[43]

ANTIHISTAMINES

First generation antihistamines such as Benadryl (diphenhydramine) and Vistaril, Atarax (hydroxyzine) easily cross the blood-brain barrier and a common side effect is sedation. The second generation drugs such as cetirizine (e.g. Zyrtec), and desloratadine (e.g. Aerius, Clarinex-D) among others, have a limited effect on the CNS due to poor blood-brain barrier transfer. Insomnia and sleepiness are rare side effects (less than 2%).[42]

ANTIEPILEPTIC DRUGS

The most common effect on sleep by the conventional (older) antiepileptic drugs is sedation. Out of the antiepileptic drugs, gabapentin (Neurontin) and pregabalin (Lyrica) are increasingly used for neuropathic pain. The following highlights their impact on sleep:

Gabapentin: sedation is commonly reported (11-18%) with decreased sleep onset latency, increased slow wave sleep (SWS), increased REM, and increased total sleep time.[43,50]

Pregabalin: Typically sedation is less prevalent (1-13%) however this number increases to 15-21% in patients with fibromyalgia. Objective findings show an increase in slow wave sleep and decreased REM.[43]

ANTIPARKINSON DRUGS

Sleep issues are very common with Parkinson's, and patients can experience insomnia, parasomnias and daytime sleepiness. This makes it difficult to know the effects of drugs on sleep. It appears that low doses of dopaminergic medications (e.g. levodopa/carbidopa) improve sleep while higher doses can worsen sleep, although influence of the disease is a significant factor.

OTHER DRUGS

Here are additional drugs that can have an impact on sleep and are relevant in clinical practice:

Corticosteroids: (Cortisol, Dexamethasone, Prednisone) They are known to disrupt sleep. In a variety of studies, corticosteroids result in marked increase in sleep disturbance and insomnia. In objective sleep studies, their use results in a marked decrease in REM sleep.[43]

Theophylline: (respiratory stimulant and bronchodilator) Disturbed sleep is a common complaint.[43]

Decongestant Agents: (Pseudoephedrine, Phenylpropanolamine) They may cause insomnia, although there are less CNS effects than ephedrine. They can cause increased wake time during sleep if taken in the evening.[43]

RECREATIONAL DRUGS

Caffeine

It goes without saying that caffeine impacts sleep. In addition to coffee, caffeine is continuing to be introduced into various food and beverage products. It has been estimated that the average adult in western societies consumes an average of 200-300 mg of caffeine daily.[51]

Caffeine usage has been shown to delay the onset of sleep, decrease slow wave sleep (SWS) and interfere with NREM sleep homeostasis.[52] It appears that REM sleep is not affected.[53]

In one study where the effects of acute caffeine consumption one hour prior to sleep were evaluated, it was confirmed that there can be a delayed sleep onset, decreased total sleep time and decreased slow wave sleep (SWS). REM sleep was not impacted.[50] Another study looked at caffeine consumption during the afternoon and evening hours and found that caffeine decreased sleep quality and melatonin secretion.[54]

It is thought that caffeine can reduce fatigue and impact sleep from its ability to inhibit the build-up of adenosine, a sleep promoting factor. Adenosine is believed to be involved in the body's sleep drive.[52]

Withdrawal from caffeine can affect one's mood and performance. One double blind, placebo-controlled study shows that chronic moderate intake (~2 cups of coffee) resulted in a withdrawal syndrome.[53]

Nicotine

Smoking's effects on general health are well known. Nicotine impacts sleep and it has been found that direct administration of nicotine in healthy non-smokers had several effects on sleep including: increasing sleep latency, increasing overall sleep time while increasing awake time after falling asleep and decreasing slow wave sleep (SWS). For chronic smokers, sleep continuity was compromised and SWS was decreased. Additionally, withdrawal from nicotine also results in sleep disturbances.[50]

Alcohol

Although alcohol is often used as a sleep aid for those struggling with their sleep, this popular substance has a number of negative effects on sleep. Those who use alcohol to fall asleep often don't realize that tolerance develops quickly. After three to five nights, the beneficial effects wear off and dosing would need to increase.[53]

Ethanol is metabolized quite quickly and is completely metabolized within 4 to 5 hours. Unfortunately, this results in rebound wakefulness in the second half of the night which leads to frequent awakenings and shallow sleep. Additionally, sleep can be disrupted from other body systems including increased heart rate, perspiration, GI complaints and headaches. [50,53]

From a sleep stage standpoint, REM sleep is affected. It will be suppressed during the first half of the night, while a REM sleep rebound will take place during the second half of the night, often leading to increased dreams and nightmares. [50,53]

Interestingly, later afternoon drinking can still impact sleep that night, including sleep disruption during the second half of the night.[53]

Key Take-Aways

- There is a strong relationship between the prevalence of disordered breathing in those taking opioids.

- The most common side effect from drugs on sleep is sedation or daytime sleepiness.

- Caffeine inhibits the build-up of adenosine which is believed to be a factor in promoting sleep drive.

- Alcohol use results in later night sleep disruption including REM rebound, shallow sleep and increased awakenings.

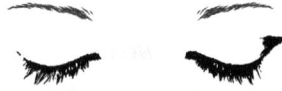

CHAPTER 4

THE DANCE BETWEEN PAIN AND SLEEP

Uncover the bidirectional relationship between sleep and pain and why it matters to your clinical practice.

COVERED IN THIS CHAPTER:
Impact of Pain on Sleep
Pain and Sleep Relationship
Additional Pain Conditions
Influence of Pain Drivers

IMPACT OF PAIN ON SLEEP

Chronic insomnia is common in those with chronic pain conditions.

As health care providers, we often interact with patients who are in pain. Pain's influence on sleep is well documented and the research shows that a majority of those suffering from chronic pain have poor sleep.

Both acute and chronic pain can influence sleep.[55] Researchers have confirmed that there is a positive correlation between pain duration and intensity, with delayed sleep onset, decreased sleep quality and fewer hours of sleep.[56] It has also been found that those who are recovering from a period of sleep deprivation will experience a temporary reduction in perceived pain.[13]

For those with chronic pain, the relationship with sleep can be a strained one. 50-70% of people with persistent pain have poor sleep quality. This number may be higher in those with fibromyalgia. It is not surprising that research has shown a positive correlation between sleep disturbance, depression and anxiety.[56]

Not only do the elderly have an increased prevalence of poor sleep quality, they are also more likely to have conditions that impact sleep. Here are a few examples:

- Arthritis and other rheumatological disorders can result in nocturnal pain and discomfort. Pain can be more noticeable at night as static postures and positions can exacerbate symptoms.

- Neuropathies such as diabetic neuropathy symptoms (e.g. burning foot pain) are typically worse at night.

- Chest and epigastric pain can be present at night from angina, reflux or peptic ulcer disease.

- Primary tumor pain is common at night.

Acute Pain

An acute injury can be an instigating factor towards the development of acute insomnia. When an injury results in an inability to find a comfortable position, patients can experience multiple awakening periods during the night. Sleep quality can deteriorate, and acute insomnia can follow. Under these circumstances, it is recommended that the patient confer with their family doctor regarding the short-term use of pain medications to help manage pain and normalize sleep patterns.

Chronic Pain

As health care practitioners, it is paramount that we understand the relationship between pain and sleep in order to truly help the patients we daily interact with.

It has been found that those with chronic pain consistently experience changes in their sleep architecture including: frequent sleep stage changes, increased nocturnal awakenings, decreased REM sleep and greater sleep fragmentation.[57]

As well, when our sleep is deprived, our ability to process nociceptive information changes. Specifically, sleep deprivation restricts select REM phases leading to a change in how our body processes nociceptive information.[17]

PAIN AND SLEEP RELATIONSHIP

Research shows that pain influences sleep and sleep influences pain.

A Bidirectional Relationship

The more you read, the more apparent the link between pain and sleep deprivation becomes. Statistics show that 50-80% of people with chronic pain have sleep dysfunction.[17]

Clinically that makes sense; people in pain are more likely to have disrupted sleep. However, the relationship between sleep and pain is more complex than this. Sleep research is beginning to uncover the more complex relationship between pain and sleep and the interaction between the two.

Newer longitudinal studies are suggesting that the causal relationship is skewed more towards the direction of sleep dysfunction increasing the risk of developing chronic pain. Currently, it's not clear whether this relationship is constant across the many different chronic pain disorders.[58]

Unfortunately, the research on understanding the relationship between sleep and pain is still very much in its infancy. Animal and human studies are limited in number and human studies are hampered by small sample sizes and lack of control groups.

In this section, I want to provide a summary of the research to date relating to sleep and pain and its implications for health care providers.

First off, I discuss the overarching view of pain, sleep and arousal. I then discuss the research surrounding the effects of acute pain on sleep including findings from both animal and human studies. I also report on the research relating to the effects of chronic pain on sleep.

Finally, I highlight the emerging research that is uncovering the powerful bidirectional nature between sleep and pain.

Pain, Sleep and Arousal

During sleep, the body is in a low state of vigilance and much of the external environment is screened out to maintain a sleep state. This process of filtering stimulus is what has been termed 'sensory gating'. When sleeping, we transition back to an awake state when sensory stimuli thresholds are surpassed.

Noxious stimuli are processed at a subconscious level when sleeping. If pain stimulus levels reach a certain level the body may experience loss of continued sleep, resulting in sleep fragmentation.[2] This fragmentation results in various attempts by our bodies to maintain sleep. Sleep fragmentation has been categorized into the following categories:

- Micro-arousals
- Awakenings
- Sleep stage shifts

These terms have been defined at the beginning of the book under Common Sleep Terms.

In sleep experiments evaluating the impact of both noxious and non-noxious stimuli across sleep stages, researchers found that although sleep was interrupted, the sleeping brain's responses varied based on the stimulus and was not uniform in nature.

It makes sense that in chronic pain, patients experience increased arousals which may interfere with falling asleep and staying asleep. In a study with fibromyalgia patients, subjects experienced more arousal episodes throughout the night as compared to healthy controls.[59]

The concept of arousal has been broadened as questions have arisen as to whether pain-related arousal is synonymous with arousal associated with chronic insomnia. As mentioned in a previous section, arousal in insomnia has been expanded to include somatic, cognitive and cortical factors. In a study with chronic pain patients, researchers found that pre-sleep cognitive arousal was a better predictor of sleep quality as compared to pain severity.[60]

However, sleep researchers argue that simply looking at arousal as the primary mechanism in disrupted sleep for pain patients is too simplistic and not sufficient to make conclusions regarding the direction of the relationship.[60,61]

Acute Experimental Pain on Sleep

A number of sleep experiments have used various noxious stimuli during various sleep stages to evaluate the effect on sleep. The main conclusions were:

- The responses are muted in comparison to a waking brain
- Sleep is disrupted (to varying degrees)
- The effects differ across the stimulus used[2]

This suggests that the brain is effective in gating sensory inputs. This gating appears to occur in brainstem sites as opposed to the cortical areas, and descending pathways may be increased during sleep.[2]

As can be expected, it is difficult to extrapolate findings from acute pain experiments in humans and animals to the more clinically relevant condition of chronic pain.

Effects of Sleep Deprivation on Pain

To better understand the relationship between sleep deprivation and pain we can look to both human and animal studies. Interestingly, animal studies focused on evaluating the impacts of REM sleep disruption while human studies focused on the effect of SWS on pain. Apparently, with rat studies it is easy to specifically disrupt REM sleep. As well, human study designs were limited given ethical considerations.

When looking at deep sleep (i.e. slow wave sleep (SWS)), 5 out of 8 studies reviewed by Lautenbacher et al showed that sleep deprivation caused hyperalgesic changes in healthy subjects.[59] It is important to note that these changes were not pathophysiological, but a direction change in pain sensitivity.

In two landmark studies conducted in 1967 by Moldofsky et al, disruption in slow wave sleep (SWS) resulted in increased myalgia pain, while disrupting REM sleep had no effect. Other studies since then have looked at disruption of SWS over three nights and found:

- Heightened somatic complaints
- Decreased pressure threshold (more sensitive to pain)
- A 'flare response' suggestive of neurogenic inflammation

The authors of the review suggest that research supports stronger sleep deprivation effects on both deep and superficial tissues (as tested with pressure pain vs temperature pain). They posit that muscle pain is influenced more by the descending pain inhibitory system and they provide support from studies that show systemic and/or widespread pain sensitivity following sleep deprivation.[61]

Although it appears that slow wave sleep (SWS) impacts pain thresholds, there is also research showing that SWS duration actually increases in the presence of pain. This is thought to be a compensation and counter-reaction to inflammation in the body.[62]

In their review of the animal sleep studies, REM sleep deprivation appears to have a hyperalgesic effect as it increased nociceptive behavior in almost all studies. As well, this REM sleep disruption appeared to block the analgesic actions of endogenous and exogenous opioids.[61]

In a 2015 meta-analysis of 34 studies evaluating the effect of sleep deprivation on pain in healthy subjects, the authors concluded that sleep deprivation increases self-reported pain and evoked pain responses with stimuli testing.[57]

Chronic Pain

It would be remiss of us to not also evaluate sleep as part of our program in helping our patients in chronic pain. This is all the more true when working with patients experiencing persistent pain. In studies where sleep quality was evaluated for patients referred to multi-disciplinary pain clinics, one study identified 70% reporting "poor sleep," while another study identified 65% classifying themselves as poor sleepers.[63]

As Smith et al succinctly states, "chronic pain may be associated with distinct physiological changes in processing of nociceptive stimuli at both central and peripheral levels as compared to acute pain." The increasing recognition of the central and peripheral systems has implications with sleep as well.[62]

In their review, they highlight some interesting findings from various clinical studies as it relates to sleep and chronic pain:

- Poor sleep can lead to increased attention to pain during the day, which can predict night-time sleep disturbance.

- Poor sleep quality and night awakenings predicted next morning pain in burn patients. However, day-time pain in these patients did not affect sleep.

- Pain and sleep disturbance were found to be predictors of long-term sleep disturbance in various studies.[62]

Neurobiological Impacts

It is possible that sleep and pain actually share common neurobiological systems, specifically central serotonergic neurotransmission which may become disrupted with pain and poor sleep.[64] It appears that limiting non-REM sleep or disrupting general sleep continuity limits the ability of the serotonergic system from functioning properly, thus impacting our bodies' opioid system and the descending inhibitory pain system.[61]

As opioid analgesia is dependent on REM sleep, sleep deprivation inhibits opioid protein synthesis and reduces the function of endogenous and exogenous opioids in the body.[59,65] This leads to an increase in self-reported pain and in pain responses with somatosensory pain testing protocols, including heat, pressure and laser pain thresholds.[57]

On the other end of the spectrum, the perception of pain stimulates arousal and leads to a release of neurochemicals associated with stress. This stress response results in disrupted sleep.[59]

Serotonin and dopamine, neurotransmitters we know play an important role in regulating the sleep/ wake cycle, may also play an important role in this bidirectional relationship. It's hypothesized that serotonergic cells involved in sleep and arousal (in the raphe nuclei) become dysregulated with chronic pain.[58,64] As serotonin dysfunction may negatively impact sleep, some studies have also found that it may lead to an increased sensitivity to thermal pain.[17] Some evidence has also found a link between dopamine levels and fibromyalgia and facial pain, however more evidence is needed to identify the exact mechanism.[58]

ADDITIONAL PAIN CONDITIONS

Be aware of certain conditions that are strongly correlated with poor sleep.

Headaches

Sleep and headaches have an interesting relationship. Sleep can be found to resolve headaches, while people can also wake up at night or in the morning with a headache. There are a number of headache disorders that involve sleep, such as various migraine types and cluster headaches, among others.[66]

There is a strong correlation between headaches and disordered sleep. A recent review of worldwide longitudinal population studies showed an increased association of 40-70% between insomnia symptoms and headaches/migraines.[67] It is reported that insomnia is the most common sleep complaint in headache clinics and may occur in more than half of patients with migraines.[68]

In one study, the following was found:

- Migraine sufferers were 3x more likely to experience excessive daytime sleepiness.
- Tension headache subjects were 3x more likely to have severe sleep disturbance (5x for migraine subjects and 17x for chronic headache subjects).[69]

For those with migraines, one study of nearly 1,300 migraine sufferers found that shortened sleep patterns were related to more frequent and severe migraines. As well, sleep disturbance and oversleeping were identified as acute triggers for migraine headache sufferers.[70]

While the underlying pathophysiology behind this relationship remains unknown, there is some evidence to suggest that awakening from slow wave sleep or experiencing REM sleep within 9 minutes of waking increases the odds of a migraine.[68] Hormone secretion levels may also play a role. There is some evidence that there is decreased hormone secretions of melatonin and prolactin in those with chronic migraine.[66]

Needless to say, the link between sleep and headaches is undeniable and worth addressing in a subjective history.

Fibromyalgia

Patients with fibromyalgia syndrome (FMS) commonly experience symptoms including sleep dysfunction, fatigue, anxiety and depression, as well as point tenderness throughout the body.[71]

Although not fully understood, the current hypothesis for the etiology of FMS is suspected to be one of central sensitization, increased peripheral nociception from wind-up, altered neurochemistry (e.g. substance P) and changes to the hypothalamus-hypophysis-adrenal axis.[72]

Sleep is a major challenge for those with FMS. Studies have shown that 94-96% of those with FMS are poor sleepers, but self-reporting within this demographic is often worse than objectively measured sleep deficits.[73]

Those with fibromyalgia often complain of: difficulty getting to sleep, struggling with multiple awakenings and experiencing unrefreshing sleep. Brainwave evaluation (EEG) has shown that those with fibromyalgia do take longer to get sleep, have extended Stage 1 sleep, have frequent arousals, and experience little slow wave sleep.[74]

What is interesting is that research is showing that disturbed sleep precedes pain in those with fibromyalgia.[74] Disrupted sleep may alter the central nervous system and actually put people at increased risk for FMS.[73]

In a longitudinal study of fibromyalgia patients, researchers found that poor sleep predicted pain and pain subsequently led to decreased physical functioning outcomes and to depression.[74]

Pharmacological and non-pharmacological treatments for FMS pain, as well as CBT and sleep hygiene education, have been shown to help manage sleep disturbance. Unfortunately, the effect of exercise is unclear.[71]

Thankfully, it appears that cognitive behavioral therapy for insomnia (CBT-I) has similarly positive effects in healthy poor sleepers as those with fibromyalgia. In a recent RCT, fibromyalgia subjects experienced improved sleep outcomes, fatigue, functional outcomes, pain catastrophizing, anxiety and depression compared to sleep hygiene education.[73]

Other Conditions To Consider

Rheumatic diseases and arthritis are common conditions health care providers see in their clinic.

In a study by Nicassio et al, 60% of people with rheumatoid arthritis (RA) reported pain interfering with sleep and 14% of those people reported the effect as severe or very severe.[75] In an earlier study, it was found that 34% of this population reported insomnia and 52% reported middle of the night awakenings.[76]

In a study with knee osteoarthritis, Campbell et al found that although a causal pathway couldn't be identified, patients with lower sleep efficiency (time asleep vs time in bed) had high central sensitization as compared to controls.[77]

Sjorgen's syndrome (a disease of the immune system where common symptoms include dry eyes and mouth) results in sleep problems. In fact, 75% of respondents with primary Sjorgens syndrome reported moderate to severe sleep disturbance.[78]

INFLUENCE OF PAIN DRIVERS

Don't underestimate the connection between depression, anxiety, insomnia and pain.

Depression and Pain

Research has shown that a significant number of people who are seeking treatment for chronic pain also have high rates of clinical depression. Research reviews highlight this number often to be over 20%.[78]

In a study looking at the combined impact of depression and insomnia on pain, researchers identified the correlation that those with major depression and insomnia also had the highest level of pain-related impairment.[79]

In evaluating the available research, researchers Boakye et al state that depression, chronic pain, and insomnia are "fundamentally interconnected" and they urge developing a unified understanding to help improve one's treatment strategy.[80]

They share a number of possible neurobiological changes that may affect those with chronic pain, depression and insomnia:

- Atrophy of the hippocampus and increased limbic area activation (the hippocampus is part of the limbic system and involved in long term memory)

- Decreased pre-frontal cortex (PFC) activity resulting in elevation of limbic activity (decreased PFC activation results in elevated limbic activity which leads to increased emotional responsiveness to circumstances)

- Dysregulation of the HPA axis leading to increased sensitivity to cortisol secretion (Cortisol is a key hormone secreted during the stress response)

- Decreases in the BDNF secretion (a growth factor that is important in brain plasticity and may play a role in the regulation of the stress response)

- Changes in the serotonergic pathways (these pathways are involved in promoting an inhibitory pain effect via the descending pathways)

- Elevated levels of pro-inflammatory cytokine release

- Decreased availability of monoamines in depression and chronic pain conditions (they are involved in the inhibitory descending pathways)

Anxiety and Pain

Anxiety is another potential pain driver. Although there are a number of anxiety conditions such as PTSD, OCD, social phobia, etc., we will focus on generalized anxiety disorder (GAD). Those with GAD are known as "pathological worriers" and controlling their worry can be a challenge. The linkage between anxiety and depression is strong.

Those with GAD are more likely to also suffer from depressive disorders and those with depression are more likely to suffer from anxiety.[81]

One may wonder about the difference between anxiety and fear. Although they are often interchanged, there is distinction. Anxiety is future focused and not linked to an observable threat, whereas fear is present focused with an avoidable observable threat.[81]

There are a number of strong connections between chronic pain and anxiety reported in a number of studies:

- Anxiety disorders were higher in people with arthritis, back pain, and migraines compared to the general population.[82]

- Those experiencing pain had a greater risk of developing first time episode of anxiety or depression.[82]

- Pain complaints are more common in people suffering with GAD than the general population.[82]

- In a study of those with arthritis, the prevalence of GAD was double that of those without arthritis (5.6% vs 2.7%).[81]

The challenge is understanding the direction of the relationship between anxiety and pain. There is limited understanding at this time of the nature of the relationship, but there is some evidence pointing to a couple of different pathways. The first is the serotonin / norepinephrine neurotransmitter system. Interestingly, drugs (e.g. SSRIs) treating this pathway can treat both anxiety and persistent pain.

Another important pathway is the hypothalamus-pituitary-adrenal (HPA) axis and its effect on corticotropin-releasing factor. Animal research has shown that elevated corticosteroids to the amygdala result in long lasting anxiety and pain.[82]

The end result of both fear and anxiety may be the same, which would include increased sympathetic nervous system (SNS) activity and amygdala activation.[81]

Overall, we see a strong relationship between anxiety, pain, depression and insomnia. Treating pain without addressing the other components may make treatment progress more difficult.

Key Take-Aways

- It's important to screen for sleep issues in those with chronic pain.

- There is a bidirectional relationship between sleep and pain and research is beginning to uncover the common shared pathways.

- Discussing sleep disturbance in patients suffering from headaches is important.

- Sleep disturbance is a hallmark challenge in those suffering with fibromyalgia and sleep disturbance has been shown to precede the development of fibromyalgia.

- There are strong connections between depression, pain and sleep and they may share common neurobiological pathways.

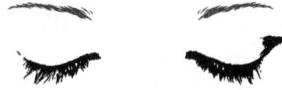

CHAPTER 5

UNDERSTANDING SLEEP SCIENCE

Understand the basics of sleep science and the key messages to share with patients.

COVERED IN THIS CHAPTER:
Sleep Cycle
Functions of Sleep
Sleep Length
Sleep Regulation
Sleep Science Patient Education

SLEEP CYCLE

The sleep cycle is a complex process that normally follows a consistent process throughout the night.

Definition of Sleep

To help our patients improve their sleep health we first need to identify the problem and understand the basics of sleep.

In its most general form, sleep can be defined as a "reversible behavioral state of perceptual disengagement from and unresponsiveness to the environment."[83] It is usually accompanied by a laying position, closed eyes, and reduction in both muscle activity and responsiveness to stimuli.[84] However, as we know, it's easy to move out of a sleep state.

There are a variety of complex physiological and behavioral processes that occur within healthy sleep that are continuing to be discovered. However, there are a variety of abnormalities that can occur with sleep such as sleepwalking, sleep talking and teeth grinding, to name just a few.[83]

The Two Basic States of Sleep

The sleep cycle is a complex process which, in healthy individuals, follows a consistent pattern. It is made up of two primary states: non-rapid eye movement (NREM) and rapid eye movement (REM). Our sleep cycle progresses from a state of wakefulness through a series of stages that involve both NREM and REM states.

We spend the large majority of our time, roughly 75-80% of our sleep, in a NREM state. It is the state where our brains and bodies are thought to be restored and recuperated.[84] While in this stage of sleep, we are considered to have relatively inactive brains in highly moveable bodies.[83]

We spend the remaining 20-25% of our sleep time in a REM state. Here, we have generalized muscle atonia with bouts of phasic muscle twitches and episodic bursts of rapid eye movement. The reduction of postural muscle tone occurs as a result of our brainstems inhibiting spinal motor neurons. It is also the state in which we dream most vividly. When you consider REM sleep, think of a highly active brain in a paralyzed body. It is also interesting to note that during the REM stage, various autonomic processes such as heart rate, blood pressure and breathing frequency vary.[85]

Normal, non-pathological sleep will begin through a NREM stage. While the specific moment of sleep onset is widely debated, many agree that sleep onset is associated with a marked reduction in skeletal muscle activity, breathing frequency, body temperature and blood pressure.[83,84] If sleep begins with REM stage sleep, it may be grounds for a diagnosis of narcolepsy (a condition characterized by uncontrolled daytime sleepiness), but we'll touch more on sleep disorders later. The following table provides a summary of the differences between NREM and REM sleep.[1,83,84,85]

NREM Sleep	REM Sleep
75-80% of sleep time	20-25% of sleep time
Relatively inactive brains in highly moveable bodies	Highly active brain in a paralyzed body
Decreases in body muscle activity, breathing frequency, heart rate, body temperature and blood pressure	Increases (and increased variability) in heart rate, breathing frequency, blood pressure and sexual arousal

NREM Sleep	REM Sleep
3 levels of NREM sleep, characterized by less short wave (alpha wave) activity and increasing slow (delta wave) wave activity	Predominantly short wave (alpha wave) activity
Brains and bodies are restored	Generalized muscle atonia with bouts of phasic muscle twitches and bursts of rapid eye movement
	Dream most actively

Understanding the Sleep Cycle

Having reviewed the two states present during sleep, we can review the sleep cycle.

Sleep moves through consistent cycles during the night with specific physiological differences in each stage. Traditionally, the sleep cycle was broken down into four progressive NREM sleep stages. However, sleep scoring guidelines were recently updated by the American Academy of Sleep Medicine (AASM) where the last two stages of NREM sleep were combined into one stage called N3. With this in mind, there are three sleep NREM sleep stages along with REM sleep. The stages progress in a cyclic fashion from wakefulness to N1, N2, N3, then returning to N2, N1 and then REM (Stage R).

The sleep cycle stages are defined by changes recorded by the electroencephalogram (EEG).[82] Different wave forms take place in each of the sleep stages, allowing sleep specialists to distinguish between the sleep stages.

The first NREM-REM cycle will last approximately 70 to 100 minutes while remaining cycles will average about 90 to 120 minutes in length.[1]

The sleep cycle is controlled by a variety of factors including the circadian rhythm and the sleep drive, as well as the secretion of hormones, such as melatonin, via the pineal gland. These processes are explained in more detail in the sleep regulation section.

THE SLEEP CYCLE

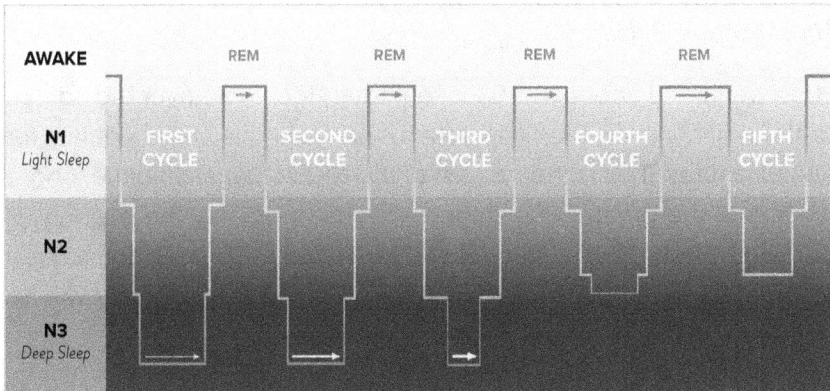

Hours progressing through the night

This diagram highlights that slow wave sleep is predominant in the earlier part of the night, while REM sleep increases in duration as the night progresses.

The Stages of Sleep

NREM Stage 1 (N1)   *Quiet Rest*

This stage acts as our transition from wakefulness to sleep. Lasting anywhere between 1-7 minutes long (approximately 2-5% of our total sleep time), one's arousal threshold is low during this stage.[83] This means that someone in stage 1 of sleep can easily be awoken. People are often not aware that they were sleeping during this state.

For people with highly disrupted sleep who wake up several times throughout the course of a night, they will spend more sleep time in this stage.[83]

This stage is characterized by a mix of brain activities with a combination of high frequencies and slower frequencies (occupy 50% of a 30 second EEG time segment).[31]

NREM Stage 2 (N2)

Here we spend about 45-55% of our total sleep time over the course of the night. During the first cycle of the night this stage will last for 10-25 minutes. This is the longest of the NREM stages and the longer we sleep, the greater this stage expands to occupy the majority of our NREM sleep. While stage 2 NREM, like stage 1, is still considered to be a state of "light" sleep, a stimulus of greater intensity will be needed to wake someone in this stage of sleep.

This stage is characterized by the presence of specific brain activity (as measured by EEG) known as sleep spindles & K complexes.[83]

NREM Stage 3 (N3)   Slow Wave Sleep (SWS)

This is the final NREM stage of sleep and is known as deep sleep. This stage occurs before we transition into REM sleep. A healthy young adult will spend 10-20% of their sleep time in this stage.[83] The deep sleep stage occurs predominantly in the earlier sleep cycles and progressively decreases through the night. Studies have shown that those with pain conditions such as fibromyalgia syndrome spend less time in this stage.[86]

This stage is characterized by:

- Slow, distinctive waves known as delta waves (slow wave sleep)
- Hypothesized that growth and repair processes take place during slow wave sleep[87]

REM Sleep (Stage R)   *Dream State*

REM Sleep stands for Rapid Eye Movement Sleep and was defined with the observation of rapid eye movement while the eyelids were closed.

REM sleep is similar to N1, but it has a different EEG pattern (i.e. jagged pattern). REM sleep typically lasts from five to thirty minutes and occupies about 20-25% of one's sleep. While NREM sleep dominates the early part of the night, REM sleep increases in duration as the night progresses. The first REM period may only last one to five minutes, and increasingly lengthen in duration as the night progress.[1]

It is characterized by:

- Bursts of rapid eye movement while eyes are closed
- Increases in middle ear muscle activity
- Increased brain activity with increased blood flow to the brain
- Suppression of muscle activity (atonia)[85]

This stage is often referred to as paradoxical sleep as it closely resembles the brain activity and body state of wakefulness, yet one is still asleep. Unlike the other stages of sleep, arousal levels in this stage vary greatly.[85]

REM sleep patterns change in those with mental health conditions. In those with depression, the REM stage of sleep changes, including a shift in REM sleep onset, duration and density.[88]

The function of REM sleep is still unclear. This stage of sleep consumes significant amounts of energy and can expend the same or more energy as waking. The evidence regarding REM sleep and memory consolidation appears conflicted. Another suggestion has been that REM sleep serves to stimulate the brain, as humans are more alert waking from REM sleep than NREM sleep.[85]

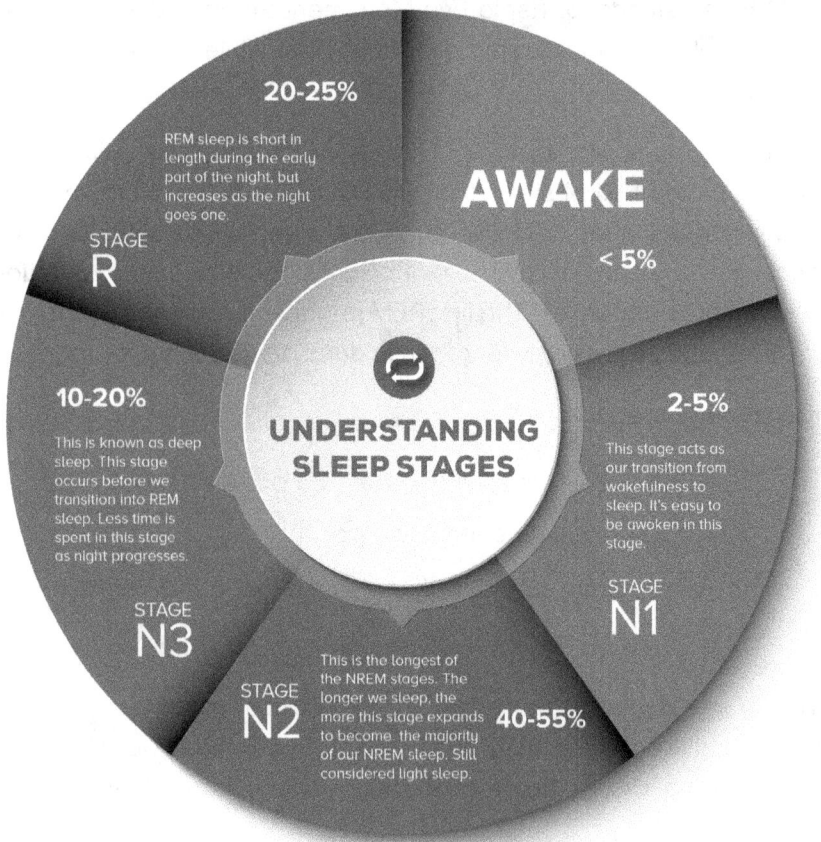

20-25%

REM sleep is short in length during the early part of the night, but increases as the night goes one.

STAGE R

AWAKE

< 5%

UNDERSTANDING SLEEP STAGES

10-20%

This is known as deep sleep. This stage occurs before we transition into REM sleep. Less time is spent in this stage as night progresses.

STAGE N3

2-5%

This stage acts as our transition from wakefulness to sleep. It's easy to be awoken in this stage.

STAGE N1

This is the longest of the NREM stages. The longer we sleep, the more this stage expands to become. the majority of our NREM sleep. Still considered light sleep.

STAGE N2

40-55%

This visual highlights the different stages of sleep along with key information associated with each stage.

FUNCTIONS OF SLEEP

Sleep's functions are complex and not yet fully understood.

It is easy to forget that there are numerous functions to sleep aside from reducing one's tiredness at the end of the day.

At this time, there is no unified understanding of sleep's function. However, there are a number of proposed theories of the functions of sleep.

Energy Conservation

Sleep appears to help conserve energy. In fact, human body and cerebral metabolic rates decrease by 15% during sleep.[84] Sleep also results in decreased motor activity and heat loss (e.g. insulation with blankets, sleep postures, piloerection) resulting in less energy expenditure. This energy conservation may help the brain and body to recuperate, although specific mechanisms are unclear.

On the contrary, it appears that the energy savings can be quite modest (80-130 calories) which doesn't appear to be much. As Lockley and Foster highlight, REM sleep may actually increase energy expenditure in contrast to the energy saving feature of NREM sleep.[3]

Oxidative Stress

During our waking state, free radical levels build up and accumulate in our bodies. In animal studies, sleep deprivation showed increased oxidative stress markers which would suggest increased production of free radicals. Although preliminary, it's possible that sleep gives the body an opportunity of decreased activity to support cell and tissue repair.[84]

Immunity

From life experience, we appreciate that sleep plays a role in supporting healthy immunity. Animal studies appear to support the idea that sleep deprivation increases susceptibility to illness and vice versa. Specifically, Peever et al share research revealing that:

- Sleep deprivation leads to increased rates of infection
- Infection results in increased NREM sleep which is hypothesized to support recuperation
- Increased mortality rates for rats experiencing sleep deprivation who had bacterial infections[84]

In humans and animals, sleep deprivation increases immune mediator levels (including leukocytes, granulocytes, monocytes). Animal research indicates that high doses of central inflammatory cytokines impaired both NREM and REM sleep.[84]

Protein Synthesis and Regulation

Another proposed function of sleep is cell regeneration. Animal studies have shown significant decreases in specific new brain cells when deprived of sleep. One process involved in the development of new brain cells is protein synthesis. It appears that protein synthesis is greater in NREM sleep and early research shows genes involved in this process are affected by sleep.[84]

Memory And Learning

We intuitively know that sleep and memory are connected. It makes sense from our own life experience that poor sleep can influence one's ability to perform newly learned tasks, recall conversations, and remember facts.

It is argued that memory formation may be sleep's most important function as it helps to establish a state of consciousness when awake.[89] Numerous studies show that newly acquired memories benefit from sleep whereby memory consolidation can take place.[90]

To begin to understand the relationship between memory and sleep, we need to review the different types of memory. Memories can be divided into:

- Declarative memories, which include events (episodic) and facts (semantic)
- Procedural memories

Another way of remembering the difference is that declarative memories are *knowing what*, while procedural memories are *knowing how*.

An important framework in understanding sleep and memory type is the dual-process hypothesis. This framework links the different sleep states with specific memory processes:

- REM sleep benefits the consolidation of procedural memories & emotional memories
- Slow Wave Sleep (SWS) benefits consolidation of declarative & spatial memories[90,91]

There appears to be sufficient evidence that sleep, especially slow wave sleep (SWS), supports the development of long term memory. Not only is this done in a passive manner (through protecting against passive interference), but it appears that sleep helps to support active consolidation through reactivating newly encoded memories in the hippocampus.[89]

The reviewed evidence shows that sleep disorders associated with increased arousal levels and disrupted sleep architecture (e.g.

insomnia, obstructive sleep apnea and narcolepsy) negatively impact the consolidation of both declarative and procedural memories.[92]

To better understand sleep's role in learning and memory, it is helpful to outline the process of memory formation. They are: encoding, consolidation and retrieval.[89] To summarize, when awake, the brain encodes memories and a memory trace is formed due to the particular stimulus.

While asleep, external stimuli to the brain is much reduced, providing an opportunity to 'consolidate' memories into long-term storage. The memory trace is reactivated and stabilized. It is believed that without sleep, recent memory traces are highly susceptible to loss.[93] Here is a helpful table to highlight the impacts of long term disrupted sleep as it relates to specific sleep stages.[91]

Sleep Stage Affected	Impact on Memory
Poor Deep Sleep (NREM 3)	More difficulty with declarative memory
Poor REM Sleep	More difficulty learning novel procedural tasks
Poor Stage 2 Sleep (NREM 2)	Difficulty performing simple motor tasks and difficulty with declarative memories
Generally Poor Sleep (all stages)	Poorer long-term memory across all memory types

There is conflicting evidence relating to the role of REM sleep in memory consolidation and certain studies have shown no negative effect with suppressing REM sleep.[85] Obviously, there is still much to be explored in sleep's role with memory and learning. Suffice it to say, sleep plays a significant role and should not be trivialized.

SLEEP LENGTH

Although the average sleep time for adults is 7-9 hours per night, it varies by individual and life stage.

There is much debate regarding the ideal length of time to sleep. While 8 hours is the most commonly cited number in the general media, studies show quite a range in the hours of sleep needed and can vary greatly across individuals.

There are many factors that can affect the amount of sleep we get at night; however, the majority of them are within our volitional control. This includes scheduled commitments, the use of an alarm clock and intentionally staying up late.[83]

When these restraints are removed and "natural" sleep is observed, the daily length of time spent sleeping is closer to 9.5 to 10 hours.[94] Sleep length can also be influenced by our genetic makeup, as well as our personal circadian rhythm.[83]

Age And Sleep

A person's stage in life is another factor that has a strong influence on our sleep cycle and quality.

Infants

Neonates spend a significant amount of time sleeping (e.g. 16 hours) with a majority of that time (50%) in REM sleep.[96] The sleep cycle in newborns differs from adults, as they can very quickly transition into REM sleep. As well, their sleep cycles are shorter; 50-60 minutes as compared to 90 minutes in young adults.[83,84]

By age two, time to REM onset will extend to 50-90 minutes and the REM cycle will begin to lengthen. Throughout the early years, sleep length will be high and REM sleep will gradually decline.[95]

Children

The amount of slow wave sleep (SWS) is greatest in young children and decreases with age. In fact, NREM sleep decreases by almost 40% at twenty years old, with continued decreases with aging. Slow wave sleep in children is different in nature than adults. Children are nearly impossible to wake while in a deep sleep. A study was conducted where 10 year-olds were exposed to 123dB tone and were not aroused![95]

Preadolescent children will decrease their sleep time from an average of 10 hours to 7.5 hours of sleep per night. Unlike adults, children at this time will rarely experience daytime sleepiness.[95]

Adolescents

In adolescence, length of time spent sleeping will suddenly increase and adolescents are less likely to be awoken during their sleep. Adolescents will also begin to experience daytime sleepiness despite this marked increase in sleep time.[95]

Adults

Sleep length studies in the UK show a range of sleep length for adults with an average of 7 hours of daily sleep, which has remained unchanged over the past 50 years.

One sleep length survey of 110,000 adults by Krueger and Friedman revealed a spread of less than 5 hours to greater than 9 hours of average sleep per night with the majority of respondents sleeping between 7 and 8 hours per night.[96]

Older Adults (>65 years)

Increased sleep disruptions become more common with age. In an American survey of 9,000 people, nearly 30% of those over 65 had problems with maintaining sleep.[97]

As noted earlier, slow wave sleep (SWS) decreases from its high in young children and continues to decrease throughout the lifespan. In fact, by 60 years of age, SWS can be significantly decreased while women appear to maintain SWS later into life.

In comparison to SWS, REM sleep remains relatively constant as a percentage of total sleep time and REM sleep has been associated with higher cognitive functioning in the older adult.[83]

Another significant change with increased age is the frequency of arousals. More frequent arousals are experienced, and it takes longer for older adults to get back to sleep.[95]

Insomnia has been shown to increase the risk for falls in the elderly. In fact, it was shown that those getting less than 5 hours of sleep had a 50% increased risk for falls.[97]

It appears, in reading about age related changes, that there is significant variability between older adults in their sleep patterns.[97] With that in mind, making broad brush strokes about age related sleep changes is difficult.

SLEEP REGULATION

Sleep regulation is controlled by sleep drive and the circadian clock.

Understanding the processes that regulate our sleep will enable us to have meaningful conversations with patients about the influences of sleep duration and quality.

The sleep regulation model proposed over 30 years ago by Borbely continues to be conceptually useful in our understanding of sleep regulation.[98]

This model consists of two primary processes:

- Sleep/Wake homeostasis (i.e. sleep homeostat)
- Circadian clock or rhythm

The first process is the sleep/wake homeostasis and is known as *Process S*. The pressure to sleep builds as the amount of time awake increases and is relieved once you sleep. Although extensively studied, this process is poorly understood.

The second process is the circadian clock or pacemaker and is known as *Process C*. It operates on a near 24-hour rhythm and is synchronized by daily environmental cues (e.g. light-dark cycle).[3]

These processes work to influence the timing as well as the duration and quality of our sleep.

Sleep Drive

Maintaining homeostasis is important for all physiological processes of the body. Like other parts of human physiology, our body works hard to maintain homeostasis between our sleep-wake cycle.

As mentioned, one process involved in sleep wake regulation is the sleep/wake homeostat (Process S), which acts as a sleep-wake "counter". It represents sleep debt which increases with hours of wakefulness and is reduced during hours of sleep. This pressure to sleep is lowest when you wake up in the morning and greatest just before bed.

This process has upper and lower bounds. When the upper bound is reached, sleep is triggered and when the lower bound is reached, awakening occurs. These oscillating upper and lower bounds correspond to a typical night and day cycle, synchronized with the circadian pacemaker.[98]

There are a number of factors that can decrease this drive to sleep which include:

- Daytime napping
- Extended sleeping (staying in bed longer)
- Consumption of caffeine
- Lack of physical activity during the day[31]

The Circadian Rhythm

Our sleep is controlled by a biological clock known as the circadian clock or pacemaker. Within the model of sleep regulation, it is referred to as Process C, which works with the sleep drive to regulate our sleep-wake cycle.

This rhythm is important in sleep-wakefulness cycles as it helps to modulate brain arousal and sleep, neurocognitive function (e.g. vigilance, cognitive speed, memory), mood and development.[36]

The primary circadian controller of the body is a group of cells located in the hypothalamus known as the suprachiasmatic nuclei (SCN).

UNDERSTANDING THE SLEEP DRIVE

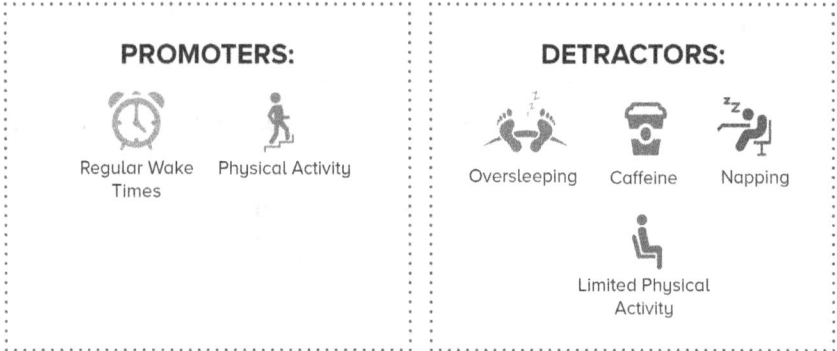

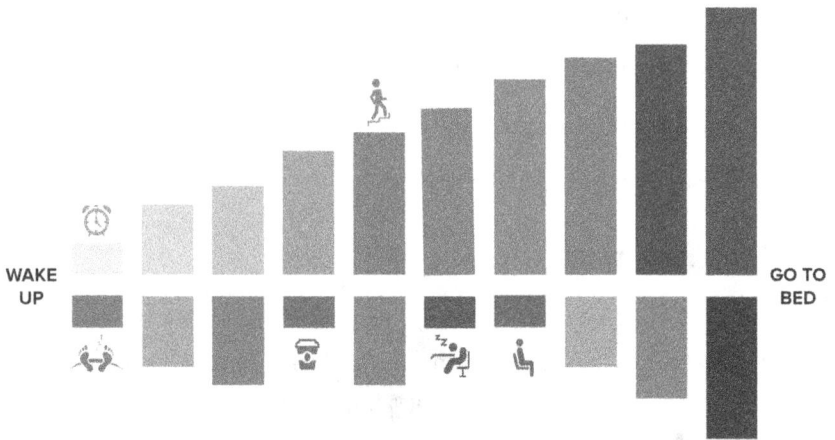

PROMOTERS:		DETRACTORS:		

PROMOTERS:

Regular Wake Times

Physical Activity

DETRACTORS:

Oversleeping

Caffeine

Napping

Limited Physical Activity

WAKE UP

GO TO BED

This visual highlights how the sleep drive is impacted by certain activities

Independent of any environmental cues, the SCN will generate near 24-hour rhythms which influences a number of body systems and processes such as temperature regulation, hormone secretions and glucose levels, among others.[3]

Our bodies look for environmental cues to maintain an accurate 24-hour cycle. The most important environmental cue is the light-dark cycle. Light captured by our eyes is transmitted via unique photoreceptors (ganglion cells) in the retina with direct connections to the SCN through the optic nerve (via the retinohypothalamic tract).[3]

Morning	Evening	Night
We wake after body temperature has reached low and begins to rise	Body temperature is at its highest and begins to drop before bedtime	Lowest body temperature occurs. Awakening occurs 1-3 hours after low
Circadian clock alerting signals rise throughout the day along with body temperature	Alerting signals begin to decrease along with lowering body temperature	Alerting signals begin to increase along with body temperature

One of the markers of the circadian rhythm is body temperature. Body temperature fluctuates in a cyclical fashion in parallel with the rising and falling of alerting signals of the circadian clock. Over a 24-hour period, the lowest temperature occurs in the middle of the night (36.5°C) and the highest temperature (37.4°C) occurs in the evening.[31]

We like to go to bed shortly after our body's temperature has peaked and begins to decrease (coincides with decreased alerting signals). We tend to wake up after about 1-3 hours after our body temperature has bottomed out which coincides with when alerting signals begin to increase.

Another important marker of Process C is melatonin. Produced in the pineal gland, melatonin is a hormone that plays a key role in the circadian rhythm.[99] Melatonin, known as the "Dracula" hormone, is secreted only at night and in the absence of light. Since it is sensitive to light, melatonin adjusts our bodies to the changing seasons.[3]

Produced by the pineal gland, melatonin output peaks between approximately 2am - 4am.[52] There is some question as to the function of melatonin, but artificial light at night increases alertness and decreases melatonin secretion.[3]

Interaction between Sleep Drive and the Circadian Rhythm

There is an interaction between Process S (sleep drive) and Process C (circadian clock). The two processes work together so that sleep can take place at night.

For example, sleep drive increases throughout the day and sleep can take place when this is high and the alerting factors from circadian clock begin to decrease.

We're able to maintain sleep throughout the night since even though our sleep drive has replenished, the alerting factors from the biological clock haven't kicked in yet. We begin to awake when those alerting signals begin to increase again.[31,100]

Disruptions to the Circadian Rhythm

This internal rhythm can be interrupted and reset by many factors such as:

- Sunlight
- Noise
- The emotional effect of social interactions

- Chemicals like caffeine, nicotine and alcohol
- The chemistry of stress and pain[36]

When this internal rhythm is disrupted and moves out of sync with one's day-night cycles, chronic sleep problems may develop. These sleep problems are called circadian rhythm sleep-wake disorders (CRSWD) and may result in cognition, learning and behavioral/emotional impairments.[35,36]

Morning and Evening Preference

People vary in terms of when they like to go to bed and wake up. There appears to be a sleep gene which influences this preference. There are two chronotypes (preferences) with sleep:

Morning Chronotype (The Lark)

- Go to bed earlier and wake up earlier
- Wake time, temperature low and melatonin rhythm occur earlier[101]
- Alertness and performance decrease quickly throughout the day[3]
- Those with insomnia fall asleep easily, but find it difficult to stay asleep[31]

Evening Chronotype (The Owl)

- Their circadian clock is delayed relative to the earth's clock resulting in delayed wake time, temperature low and melatonin rhythm[31, 101]
- Difficulty waking at normal times and takes longer to feel alert after waking
- For those with insomnia they may have difficulty falling asleep, and maintaining sleep in first part of the night[31]

UNDERSTANDING
THE CIRCADIAN RHYTHM

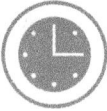

A CLOCK THAT DOESN'T STOP

It helps to regulate our sleep cycle and is based on a 24-hour clock.

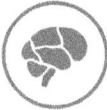

SCN BRAIN CELLS

A group of cells in our brain keep our 24-hour cycle going. This is the primary control center for this rhythm.

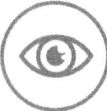

LIGHT-DARK CYCLE

This fine tunes our 24-hour cycle. It influences our sleep cycle. Melatonin only gets released when it's dark.

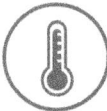

BODY TEMPERATURE

This fluctuates over a 24-hour period. We sleep best when body temperature begins to drop.

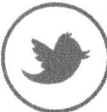

PERSONAL PREFERENCE

Each person has a preference: Morning Lark or Night Owl.

This visual highlights highlights the key patient messages regarding the circadian rhythm.

Sleep Debt

If insufficient sleep is had, the sleep drive cannot be properly replenished which will lead to a "sleep debt". Sleep debt is repaid with an increased intensity and duration of subsequent NREM sleep. The change to REM sleep under these circumstances will be very minimal. This concept of sleep debt can also be applied to too much sleep. Under these circumstances the need for sleep will be reduced.[84]

Sleep debt is simply the difference (deficit) between a person's ideal amount of sleep for optimal functioning and the amount of sleep they actually receive.[102] In other words:

Sleep Debt = Ideal Sleep Time vs Actual Sleep

The consequence and the primary sign of sleep debt is excessive daytime sleepiness (EDS). Sleepiness can be measured using various finely tuned lab instrumentation. However, sleep researchers Horne and Burley believe that people can be good detectors of their own sleepiness simply by allowing themselves to settle down and relax and then evaluating their sleepiness.[96]

Research evaluating ideal sleep times suggests that there is a fair amount of variability between individuals. Sleep length studies show a range of sleep length for individuals with an average of 7 hours daily sleep. This has remained unchanged over the past 50 years. As previously mentioned, a large sleep length survey found a spread of less than 5 hours to greater than 9 hours of average sleep per night with most people sleeping between 7 and 8 hours per night.[96]

Although the research is conflicting, it appears that adapting to shorter sleep duration can be safely done without negative impacts. Horne has proposed that an adaptable range of safe sleep is between 6 to 9 hours per day.[96]

Although there is a certain amount of flexibility with sleep length, chronic under-sleep has an impact. With both physical and mental health consequences, it can result in appetite, mood and depressive symptoms and an increase in morbidity and mortality.[96,102]

Thankfully, sleep debt can be repaid with short, timely naps. Short naps (less than 20 minutes) can be as effective as extending nightly sleep by one hour.[103] This finding should be tempered with the understanding that while napping can be helpful for healthy sleepers, it can have a significant negative effect for poor sleepers due to the impact on the sleep drive.

SLEEP SCIENCE PATIENT EDUCATION

4 Key Principles to Empower Your Patients

Empower Your Patients

Explaining the basics of sleep to patients can lay some important groundwork for helping them with their sleep, and thus helping them with their overall health.

First, by empowering patients with an understanding of how their body works, you equip them with the knowledge to change their behavior and habits. The better they understand the "why," the greater chance they have of staying motivated to make the necessary lifestyle and environmental changes.

Second, a patient's understanding of the sleep cycle will help them decipher their own, should they choose to use specific activity and sleep trackers.

4 Key Principles for Patients

After my research and review of the science of sleep, I believe there are four key educational messages for patients when discussing the sleep basics:

1: Sleep Length Varies by Person

The adage that we need 8 hours of sleep may be a good general guideline, but can cause anxiety for those who sleep less. Explaining the variability that exists in sleep length across individuals, along with the changes that take place as we age, can help to reduce that anxiety.

2: A Healthy Sleep Cycle is a Must for Sleep Health

By having patients understand the sleep cycle, they can understand the importance of experiencing the different stages of sleep. Healthy sleep can vary between individuals, but should follow the basic sleep cycle. Although objective measurement is needed to properly evaluate the quality of the sleep cycle, there are indicators of good sleep that patients can make note of. These include:

- Few night awakenings
- Minimal restlessness during sleep
- Feeling refreshed upon waking
- Healthy daytime functioning

3: A Healthy Sleep Cycle Requires a Consistent Circadian Rhythm

To ensure a healthy sleep cycle, one must respect and support a consistent circadian rhythm. Patients need to understand that variable wake times impact the body's circadian rhythm. This rhythm is easily influenced by environmental and behavioral factors and is under the patient's control.

4: Your Sleep Drive Must Be Respected

By educating patients on the importance of the deep sleep drive, patients can better understand why regular sleep times and sleep efficiency is so important.

The sleep drive is easily impacted (and negatively affected) by daytime napping, limited physical activity and spending too long in bed. Better quality sleep can be achieved by educating patients on the sleep drive and the importance of delaying bedtime until their drive to sleep is strong.

These principles will likely need to be reinforced and reviewed with patients as they are easy to forget in our highly stimulating, technology driven world.

4 KEY PRINCIPLES TO HEALTHY SLEEP

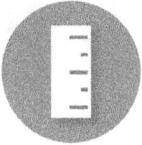

SLEEP LENGTH VARIES BY PERSON & AGE
Understand what works for you. Normal sleep length can range from 6 to 9 hours and it's important to know your optimal number.

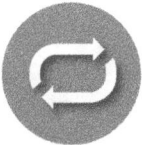

A HEALTHY SLEEP CYCLE IS NEEDED FOR REFRESHING SLEEP
You can't cheat your body's sleep cycle. Trying to boost your performance in life shouldn't come at the expense of the regular sleep cycle.

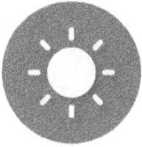

STRENGTHEN YOUR CIRCADIAN RHYTHM
Consistency is key. Get up at the same time every day. This will create a deeper anchor to strengthen your sleep cycle. Don't forget to decrease artificial light well before bed.

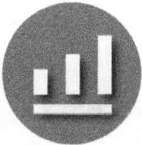

DO THINGS THAT BUILD YOUR SLEEP DRIVE
Engage in activities and behaviours that build your pressure to sleep. The stronger this drive, the easier it will be to fall asleep and stay asleep.

This visual highlights the key principles to healthy sleep to reinforce with patients.

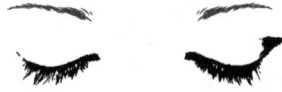

CHAPTER 6

EVALUATING SLEEP HEALTH

Become familiar with the key evaluation tools and strategies in evaluating disrupted sleep.

COVERED IN THIS CHAPTER:

Subjective and Objective Evaluation

Evaluating Depression

Evaluation in the Clinic

Sleep Study Referrals

SUBJECTIVE AND OBJECTIVE EVALUATION

There are a variety of sleep measures that can help identify and measure disrupted sleep behaviors and beliefs.

Subjective Evaluation

There are a number of subjective patient report measures that can be used in the clinic to help gain a better understanding of a patient's sleep quality, beliefs and hygiene. Below, I outline the most common outcome measures found within sleep medicine.

Pittsburgh Sleep Quality Index (PSQI)

The Pittsburgh Sleep Quality Index, otherwise known as the PSQI, is the most commonly used generic sleep outcome measure.[104] Developed with no specific population in mind, it seeks to identify good sleepers and bad sleepers, and not to make a specific diagnosis. Retrospective in nature, it asks questions relating to sleep latency, sleep duration, sleep efficiency, sleep quality, sleep disturbances, medication use and daytime dysfunction over the past month. Key elements of the measure include:

- It is administered to a patient and their bed partner. There are a total of 19 self-rated questions with five questions rated by the bed partner.

- Questions are grouped into seven component scores each weighted equally (0-3 scale). The component scores are added for a global PSQI score out of 21.

- A high score signifies poor sleep quality. A global score greater than 5 resulted in sensitivity of 89% and specificity of 86% in identifying good vs poor sleepers.[105]

It is important to note that the PSQI can be a little cumbersome to score given the scoring of multiple components of sleep function and the need for partner input.

Medical Outcomes Study Sleep Scale (MOS)

Another popular outcome measure is the Medical Outcomes Study Sleep Scale (MOS). It has a total of 12 items and measures:

- Sleep quantity
- Sleep quality
- Sleep disturbance
- Daytime somnolence
- Snoring
- Respiratory problems / shortness of breath

This outcome measure has been validated in neuropathic pain and according to Cole et al is the best measure to use for patients with pain. The researchers also point out a couple of specific advantages over the PSQI:

- It provides a validated dimension and scoring for the individual element of sleep disturbance, which is a key domain for patients with pain.
- The measure is shorter to administer (12 items vs 19 items) and doesn't require a bed partner's input.[106]

The measure has good reliability and reproducibility.

Epworth Sleepiness Scale (ESS)

The gold standard for measuring daytime sleepiness is the multiple sleep latency test (MSLT). Unfortunately, it's time intensive as it takes all day for both the tester and the patient. The ESS was developed as a brief, 8 item self-administered questionnaire measuring a patient's level of daytime sleepiness. It shows significant correlation with sleep latency as measured by the MSLT during the day and at night with polysomnography.[107]

Insomnia Severity Index (ISI)

According to a research study evaluating sleep measures, Smith & Wegener indicated that the ISI is a validated, reliable and responsive screening tool for evaluating the severity of insomnia. It has been validated across both prospective sleep diary measures and polysomnographic testing.[108]

It consists of 7 items measuring perceived insomnia severity. With a potential total score of 28, the higher the score, the more severe the perceived insomnia. Using a 4-point scale it evaluates perceived severity relating to:

- Sleep onset
- Sleep maintenance
- Early morning awakening problems
- Satisfaction with current sleep pattern
- Interference with daily functioning
- Noticeable impairments attributed to the sleep problem
- Level of distress caused by sleep problem[109]

Sleep Diary

A sleep diary is a mandatory evaluation tool used in evaluating and treating insomnia and is considered the gold standard in subject sleep evaluation.[110]

A patient simply maintains a record of their daily sleep behaviors and lifestyle choices over a period of 2 weeks and can include: medications, alcohol use, caffeinated drinks, meals, exercise, mood on arising, bedtime/ arising times, awakenings, total sleep time, napping and sleep efficiency.[111]

A sleep diary helps individuals become more aware of their sleep behaviors and is an important tool in monitoring compliance with sleep hygiene interventions.

One of the challenges with sleep diaries is the multiple versions that exist. Efforts have been made to standardize the sleep diary through the development of the Consensus Sleep Diary (CSD). A few different variations were developed to gather additional information to be completed in the morning or evening. The Core Consensus Sleep Diary (CCSD) consists of 9 items that allow one full week to be printed off on one page.[110]

Dysfunctional Beliefs and Attitudes about Sleep (DBAS)

The Dysfunctional Beliefs and Attitudes about Sleep (DBAS) is a well-used instrument to evaluate disruptive sleep beliefs consisting of 30 items, with a shorter version created known as the DBAS-16.

The DBAS has been found to be reliable in distinguishing between self-described good and poor sleepers in both younger and older adults. The DBAS-16 has been shown to have adequate psychometric qualities and is a tool that is less cumbersome to use in practice.[112]

This outcome measure addresses the following domains regarding sleep beliefs and attitudes:

- Consequences of poor sleep (e.g. I cannot function without a good night's sleep)

- Worry/Helplessness (e.g. Sleep is unpredictable)

- Expectations (e.g. I need 8 hours of sleep)

- Medication (e.g. Medication is the only solution)

In evaluating a patient's response to the items, the higher the score, the greater the endorsed belief. Scoring is based on adding the scores for all 16 items and dividing by 16 for the average total score.[112]

This outcome measure can be an effective tool to guide a clinician's discussion with patients about potentially problematic beliefs.[112]

Other Measures

There are a number of other sleep measures that were mentioned in the literature, but unfortunately we were unable to find additional information. They include the following:

- Stanford Sleepiness Scale

- Toronto Sleepiness Scale

- Canadian Sleep Society Inventory

- Sleep Problem Scale

- Montefiore Sleep Questionnaire

Summary of Key Outcome Measures

Outcome Measure	Target Population	# of Items
Pittsburgh Sleep Quality Index (PSQI)	General	19 + 5 for partner
Medical Outcomes Study Sleep Scale (MOS)	Neuropathic Pain	12
Insomnia Severity Index (ISI)	General	7

Outcome Measure	Target Population	# of Items
Consensus Sleep Diary (CSD)	General	9
Dysfunctional Beliefs & Attitudes about Sleep (DBAS-16)	General	16

Objective Measures

More involved objective assessments of sleep involve three primary testing measures which are described below.

Polysomnography (PSG)

This is the gold standard objective measure to evaluate sleep related breathing disorders. It measures brain activity (EEG), eye movement (electrooculography) and muscle activity (electromyography). The testing takes place in a sleep lab.

PSG is used to identify the severity of obstructive sleep apnea syndrome (OSAS), as well as other concurrent sleep disorders.

I discovered that this method is used sparingly due to its complexity.

There are three levels of sleep studies that exist:

> **Level 1:** Polysomnography (No Level 2)

> **Level 3:** Overnight at home sleep study. Oxygen levels, heart rate, airflow, snoring and other parameters are measured.

> **Level 4:** Sleep Apnea Screening with oximetry.

Multiple Sleep Latency Test (MSLT)

The multiple sleep latency test (MSLT), as previously mentioned, is the gold standard for measuring daytime sleepiness as well as well as abnormal REM sleep onset.[113] Typically, the MSLT is performed following a night with PSG, as well as completion of a sleep diary for one to two weeks. Testing takes an entire day.

The goal of the testing is to measure the speed of falling asleep during the day in a sleep inducing environment. Using two-hour intervals, the patient is asked to lie down and recordings are taken to see how quickly sleep occurs within a twenty minute period. This process is repeated every two hours for a minimum of four periods.[113]

Actigraphy

This evaluation measures movement during sleep, sleep time, sleep efficiency and sleep disturbance. It separates a patient's sleep from wakefulness. This objective testing is less expensive and has a high level of agreement with PSG.[114] Measurements take place over several days which reduces measurement error and improves reliability. As well, the testing can be done at home.

Actigraphy shows reasonable validity and reliability in assessing sleep vs. wake patterns in normal people with average or good sleep quality. Unfortunately, actigraphy is less effective with special populations such as the elderly, children, people with major health problems and poor sleepers, due to a poor ability to detect wakefulness periods during sleep.[114]

Actigraphy is sensitive enough to detect changes in sleep from pharmacological and non-pharmacological (e.g. CBT) interventions.[114] The primary limitation with actigraphy is that it difficult to detect sleep onset timing.[55]

EVALUATING DEPRESSION

Depression is an important orange flag to identify in clinical practice.

For those of us who are direct-access health care providers, we have the privilege that allows patients to see us without referral.

With this in mind, it is important that we screen for other medical issues that may require further care or may impede their overall health.

Patients who experience low back pain have poorer outcomes if depression is present. If this is the case, then it's worthwhile to ask how good we are in identifying depression in patients with low back pain. In a study of 68 physiotherapists, researchers discovered that even though 40% of patients had depressive symptoms, the therapists were poor in their ability to identify patients with depressive symptoms.[115]

The authors of this study recommend using a simple two question screening (which fared much better than therapists) to identify depressive symptoms in patients. They are:

1. During the past month, have you often been bothered by feeling down, depressed, or hopeless?

2. During the past month, have you often been bothered by little interest or pleasure in doing things?

They recommend that if answered positively, the therapist should monitor progress closely, and if not improving, assess further with the use of the DASS-21 (see below). They then recommend that if they score moderately or severely on the DASS-21 that patients be referred for psychological evaluation and support.[115]

DASS-21

The DASS-21 is a shortened version of the original 42 item DASS measure. It's a self-report questionnaire that aims to measure the severity of a range of symptoms relating to depression and anxiety.[115]

EVALUATION IN THE CLINIC

Begin with simple questioning about sleep and use additional sleep outcome measures to explore sleep challenges.

Clinical Evaluation

It's great to have an overview of the different evaluation tools that can be used in understanding sleep dysfunction in patients. However, the challenge is how to put this into practice. Since our time with patients is limited, it's important to be selective in the outcome measures used.

Patient History

In our history taking, I believe that sleep screening should be done with every patient experiencing persistent pain and those who are at risk for disrupted sleep. A simple two question screening process will be enough to better understand if further evaluation is needed. By asking patients the following two questions, clinicians can quickly identify the need for further evaluation:

- Do you have difficulty initiating or maintaining sleep or experience early morning awakenings?
- Do you experience non-restorative sleep?[116]

SLEEP SCREENING QUESTIONS

DO YOU HAVE DIFFICULTY WITH:

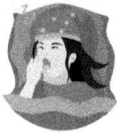

Getting to Sleep?

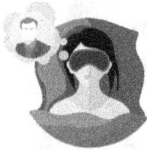

Staying Asleep?

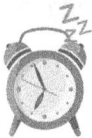

Early Wake-ups?

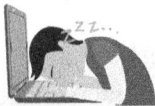

Non-Restorative Sleep?
(Feel unrefreshed, sleepy during the day)

This visual highlights the key questions to ask patients regarding their sleep.

If, in your conversation with the patient, you suspect potential sleep issues, it is worthwhile to use a comprehensive sleep screening tool such as the PSQI or the ISI. The PSQI is a great choice as it covers so many different facets of one's sleep patterns which can help guide your patient discussion and treatment planning.

During your conversation, you may discover that a patient's beliefs about sleep and sleep health may be in question. In that event, the DBAS-16 would be a useful outcome measure to use in identifying and guiding conversation about sleep beliefs and practices.

As mentioned earlier, the sleep diary is an essential tool in understanding one's sleep habits and patterns. It's easy for anyone to reflect only on their most recent night or two of sleep when reviewing sleep quality. However, tracking one's sleep patterns over a period of two weeks using the Consensus Sleep Diary is necessary. It is recommended that you, as a healthcare provider, use a sleep diary in order to experience what is involved in completing the diary. This will improve your ability to help your patients use this tool.

It is not uncommon for those with chronic sleep problems to also have issues with depression and anxiety. A simple screening questionnaire can help you determine if depression can be a concomitant issue.

As previously mentioned, the following two questions have been shown to be effective in helping physiotherapists identify depression in patients:

1. During the past month, have you often been bothered by *feeling down, depressed, or hopeless?*

2. During the past month, have you often been bothered by *little interest or pleasure* in doing things?

If patients respond in the affirmative to the above questions, the study authors recommended the use of a more comprehensive depression screening tool such as the DASS-21 or the Distress and Risk Assessment Method (DRAM).[115]

Obstructive Sleep Apnea

As previously mentioned obstructive sleep apnea (OSA) is the most common breathing problem in sleep and is severely under-diagnosed.

Although polysomnography is the gold standard for assessing for OSA, there can often be long wait times which delays proper medical care. To help improve screening for OSA, researchers Chung et al developed the STOP-Bang outcome measure which combines survey questions and other relevant items (i.e. age, BMI, gender, neck circumference).[32] The sensitivity and specificity were more than 90% for those with moderate and severe OSA. Given the effectiveness of this tool, it is recommended that this be included in the evaluation of every patient who struggles with sleep.

The **STOP** component involves the following questions:

1. Do you **s**nore loudly, (louder than talking or loud enough to be heard through closed doors)? Y/N

2. Do you feel **t**ired, fatigued or sleepy during daytime? Y/N

3. Has anyone **o**bserved you stop breathing during your sleep? Y/N

4. Do you have high blood **p**ressure? Y/N

The **Bang** component:

1. **B**MI: Is their BMI over 35 kg/m^2? Y/N

2. **A**ge: Are they over 50 years old?

3. **N**eck: Is their neck circumference more than 40 cm or 15 inches? Y/N

4. **G**ender: Are they male? Y/N

High Risk for OSA: Yes to 3 or more questions

Low Risk for OSA: Yes to less than 3 questions

During the physical exam, it is helpful to make note of patient obesity, neck girth, signs of depression and apical breathing patterns. These physical signs help in better understanding the presence of sleep apnea.

Screening for sleep apnea is important in identifying the need for further medical evaluation and treatment, including referral to a sleep specialist.

SLEEP STUDY REFERRALS

Sleep studies are not routinely recommended for insomnia unless there are other issues present.

It can be challenging to know when a patient should be referred for a sleep study. Access to sleep specialists is limited and wait times can be long depending on the availability of sleep specialists in the specific city or region. In Canada, the average wait time to access a sleep study is approximately four to six months.[117] It is important to identify the wait times in your local area as they can vary.

With this in mind, it's important as health care providers to understand when to request that a family physician refer a patient for a sleep study.

According to the American Academy of Sleep Medicine (AASM), sleep studies are not routinely recommended unless there are co-morbid conditions or other sleep disorders present.[118]

Physicians are encouraged to request polysomnography when the following are present:

- Suspected breathing (e.g. sleep apnea) or movement disorders
- Uncertain diagnosis
- Behavioral and/or pharmacological treatment is not effective
- Violent or injurious behaviors as a result of "precipitous arousals"

Actigraphy evaluation can be helpful in quantifying circadian rhythms patterns or sleep disturbances.[118]

Sleep Apnea

As previously mentioned, the use of the STOP-Bang is an effective screening tool for sleep apnea. It is recommended that if a patient has a score greater than three, they should be referred to their family doctor for further evaluation in potentially having obstructive sleep apnea (OSA).

The gold standard for diagnosing sleep apnea is polysomnography (PSG) which must be completed in a sleep laboratory.[119]

Treatment for obstructive sleep apnea consists of the following:

- **CPAP (continuous positive airway pressure):** this pressurizes the upper airway to prevent collapse during sleep
- **Oral appliance therapy:** the aim is to advance the mandible and can be considered for mild to moderate OSA
- **Bariatric surgery:** reducing weight has been shown to improve or resolve OSA

- **Nasal expiratory positive pressure (nEPAP):** the use of a small valve taped to the nostrils provides positive pressure during expiration

- **Upper airway surgery:** this includes nasal septoplasty, uvulopalatopharyngoplasty (UPPP), tonsillectomy, tongue advancement surgery, maxillomandibular advancement[121]

Key Take-Aways

- There are a number of different subjective evaluation screening tools and it's important to use a tool that best fits your patient population and clinical environment.

- The sleep diary is a mandatory sleep evaluation tool when evaluating sleep.

- Polysomnography is the gold standard for measuring sleep but is typically not needed unless other co-morbid conditions are suspected.

- Screening for the presence of sleep disruption and depression can be done by asking a few simple questions.

- Obstructive sleep apnea is often undiagnosed, and the STOP-Bang is an effective screening tool to be used in a clinical setting.

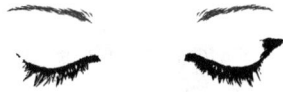

CHAPTER 7

INSOMNIA MANAGEMENT

Understand typical sleep medications, the evidence for sleep hygiene recommendations and popular alternative therapies.

COVERED IN THIS CHAPTER:
Overview
Sleep Hygiene
Exercise
Mind-Body Therapies
Other Therapies
Supplements

OVERVIEW

Sleep medications are a common intervention for insomnia, but they don't address the underlying causes of insomnia.

Pharmacology's role in treating insomnia has continued to evolve over the decades.

Prior to the 1900's, opioids, bromide salts, herbal preparations and alcohol were the main hypnotic choices for disrupted sleep. In the first half of the 20th century, barbiturates (drugs ending in barbital) were the treatment of choice but were curtailed due to their adverse effects and risk of lethal overdose.[7]

In the 1960's & 1970's, benzodiazapines (BZD) such as Librium and Valium were introduced and became popular replacements to barbiturates. There were concerns of dependency and tolerance with BZD drugs which resulted in a general decrease (1% decrease) in hypnotic prescriptions from 1970-1990. With these concerns in mind, doctors turned to sedating anti-depressants (e.g. trazadone) for the treatment of insomnia, even though studies were limited.[7]

In the 1990's, nonbenzodiazpine (non-BZD) hypnotics were introduced, including Ambien (Zolpidem). Ambien has become the most widely prescribed hypnotic medication and accounts for nearly 90% of all non-BZD prescriptions.[7]

Since 2005 additional sleep medications have been introduced to the marketplace including:

- Melatonin Agonist: Rozerem (ramelteon)
- Sedating Tricyclic Anti-Depressants: Sinequan/Silenor (doxepin)
- Orexin receptor antagonist: Belsomra (suvorexant)[7]

Common Sleep Hypnotics

Benzodiazepine Hypnotics:

Benzodiazepines affect GABA receptors in a non-specific way and produce additional effects beyond improved sleep including: daytime sedation, dizziness, lightheadedness, anterograde amnesia, motor incoordination and falls.[116,118] Respiratory depression can also be a problem in those with breathing problems (e.g. obstructive sleep apnea). There is increased risk for abuse and dependence with this class of drugs.[116]

Drug Name	Common Brand Names
Temazepam	Restoril
Estazolam	ProSom
Triazolam	Halicon
Flurazepam	Dalmane
Quazepam	Doral

Non-benzodiazepine Hypnotics:

This newer class of hypnotics tends to have fewer side effects than the above mentioned category because it has a more direct influence on certain GABA receptors. They can help decrease sleep latency and increase total sleep time.

Drug Name	Common Brand Names
Zolpidem	Ambien
Eszopiclone	Lunesta
Zaleplon	Sonata
Zopiclone	Imovane

There is less risk of abuse with these drugs but can result in the following adverse reactions: disorientation, residual sedation, nausea, nightmares, amnesia, mood changes, headache and vertigo.[116]

It is important to note that benzodiazepine hypnotics are generally well tolerated and adverse events are typically associated with increased dosing.[120]

Sleep Medication Usage

Although the risk profiles of sleep medications have been improving, the risk of dependency, tolerance and side effects are still a concern. This continues to drive the development of medications with less adverse side effects and improved efficacy.

Although the use of sleep hypnotics decreased from the 1970s to 1990s, their use is still prevalent. In the USA, 6-10% of adults were found to use hypnotic medications in 2010. In Australia, 90% of primary care interactions for insomnia led to the prescription of hypnotic medications.[121]

Hypnotics and Older Adults

The adverse event profile with sleep medications is more significant for the elderly. In a study by Singh et al, pharmacological intervention for insomnia and depression lead to a greater number of side effects in the elderly, increasing the likelihood of falls and confusion.[10] The American Geriatric Society has recommended that hypnotics, specifically benzodiazepines, are avoided in older patients due to the risk of fall, motor vehicle accidents and cognitive impairment.[7]

Canadian organizations including the: Canadian Geriatrics Society, Canadian Society of Hospital Medicine, Canadian Psychiatric societies, including Canadian Academy of Geriatric Psychiatry (CAGP) and Canadian Psychiatric Association (CPA), discourage the use of hypnotic-sedatives as a first choice in older adults according to Insomnia in adults.[122]

Effectiveness of Sleep Medication

The big question is how effective are sleep medications in improving disrupted sleep?

The AASM has outlined that hypnotic medications are as effective as CBT-I during acute treatment. However, the gains achieved from sleep medications decreased after treatment, while the gains associated with cognitive behavioral therapy for insomnia (CBT-I) continue once treatment is completed.[7]

Indications for Sleep Medications

Generally speaking, the benefit of medications is their widespread availability and when effective, rapid improvement in symptoms. However, medications have side effects, and can result in dependence and tolerance over time. The problem is that medications are not curative, so long-term use is often needed. Currently there is little evidence suggesting their efficacy and safety for use greater than one to two years.[123]

Guidelines produced for the American Academy of Sleep Medicine (AASM) acknowledge at the outset of their clinical guidelines that cognitive behavioral therapy for insomnia (CBT-I), which will be covered in a later chapter, is the standard of treatment for insomnia and should be the first line of treatment for those with chronic insomnia. However, they acknowledge that there are patients who may not benefit from CBT-I including those who:

- Are unable to access CBT-I treatment because of availability, cost, etc.

- Are unable or unwilling to participate in CBT-I therapy
- Do not respond to treatment[7]

Non-Pharmacological Interventions

We have to remember that sleep is a behavior, specifically, a learned behavior. Thankfully, as humans we have the ability to change learned behaviors.

As one can imagine, providing sedative medications to help address insomnia in chronic pain patients does not address the functional impairments such as maladaptive behaviors and beliefs causing the insomnia.[124]

Sleep hygiene rules, made popular in mainstream media, has been shown to have little effect as a stand-alone treatment for those suffering from insomnia. [125]

Before we go through the various non-pharmacological options for insomnia management, it is important to understand that the evidence is clear regarding the first line of treatment for insomnia. It should be cognitive behavioral therapy for insomnia (CBT-I). Newly published guidelines by the Academy of Sleep Medicine (AASM) for pharmacologic treatment of insomnia state that the first line of treatment for those with insomnia should be CBT-I.[7]

SLEEP HYGIENE

The evidence for sleep hygiene is limited and sleep hygiene is not enough to help those who struggle with sleep.

Overview

Sleep hygiene helps set the foundation for healthy, restful sleep.

Sleep hygiene is the staple of advice given to those struggling with sleep. It's been popularized in mainstream media and is often the first line of education. Even though sleep hygiene is promoted as a cure for insomnia in popular media we have to recognize the limitations of sleep hygiene. Sleep hygiene is helpful in setting the foundation for healthy behaviors and a sleep environment conducive to restful sleep.

Sleep hygiene can be defined as specific strategies and behavioral changes that people can make to their lifestyle and environment with the goal of improving their sleep quality. This can include addressing habits that can impact sleep such as caffeine and tobacco, as well as environmental factors such as excess light and use of electronics.

Although research is limited, it appears that in the elderly, improvements were seen in sleep latency, continuity, duration and waking moods when engaging in healthy sleep hygiene.[126]

As mentioned in the previous section, sleep hygiene is not effective in helping those struggling with chronic insomnia. It simply is not enough, and more intensive behavioral treatment is required.[127]

A question that you may be asking is, "What does sleep hygiene actually consist of?" I'm sure that in a room of 20 people we would have some common rules, but also a fair amount of variety.

Sleep hygiene rules were originally codified by Peter Hauri in the 1970's. This list was based on scientific studies (e.g. effects of caffeine and alcohol) and his own clinical experience working with those suffering from insomnia.

Unfortunately, the consistency across sleep hygiene is poor. There is no agreed upon list of rules and none of the published sleep hygiene rules have been found to be the same. In fact, out of 19 sleep hygiene rules across five different sleep hygiene lists, only six were described in at least four out of the five reviewed publications.[128]

Sleep hygiene rules can be broken down into various categories. In evaluating common themes across 19 sleep hygiene rules from five different publications, Peter Hauri identified these themes:

- Review of sleep environment
- Rules about bedtime and wake times
- Evening activities that help with sleep
- Intake before bedtime
- Attitudes during the night[125]

From the publications reviewed, Hauri identified only six hygiene rules that were consistently presented across the majority (4 out of 5) of reviewed sleep hygiene publications. They were:

- Eliminate bedroom noise
- Curtail or eliminate napping
- Exercise
- Limit or avoid caffeine
- Avoid alcohol, especially during evening
- Eat a light snack before bedtime

Below we go through a comprehensive list of sleep hygiene recommendations divided into environmental and lifestyle factors.

Environmental Factors

Eliminate Bedroom Noise

A quiet sleep environment is necessary in supporting sustained sleep. People sleep better when there is no disruptive noise. Even though we adjust to background noises, a study from Globus and colleagues discovered that people living near an airport still had disruptive sleep after 6 years.[125]

Ear plugs can be an effective strategy to block noise as can soothing, consistent background noise. White noise generators, air conditioning units or fans can all be effective tools in providing a consistent sound background.

Keep the Bedroom Dark

If we recall in our discussion of sleep regulation, the secretion of melatonin is dependent on darkness. Keeping the room dark through black-out curtains or an eye mask is important.

Keep the Bedroom Cool

A requirement for sleep is a decrease in body temperature. A room that is too warm will prevent this drop in body temperature. It appears that body temperature can decrease more quickly in a cooler room and the cooler the room, the greater the drop in body temperature.[129] Preferred temperature can vary though by person, but generally a slightly lower than daytime temperature is recommended (16-17°C seems to be optimal).[125]

Limit Bedroom Activities to Sleep and Sex

Engaging in activities *outside of* sleep and sex in the bedroom sets up maladaptive sleep conditioning. Pairing sleep and the bedroom is an important component that is discussed in a later chapter. It is generally agreed that technology such as TVs, video games and so forth should be removed from the bedroom.

Make Sure Your Bed is Comfortable

A comfortable, supportive bed can help one to sleep more soundly and avoid body aches associated with poor positioning. Another important factor is the influence of a sleeping partner in bed. Sleeping with a partner results in decreased deep sleep and decreased REM.[125]

Eliminate the Bedroom Clock

This an interesting recommendation. Peter Hauri highlighted that many insomniacs can pay too much attention to their clocks and find themselves more anxious as the minutes and hours slip by without sleep. Removing a clock helps poor sleepers from being reminded of the amount of time they are spending in bed awake and reduces a significant potential stressor.[125]

Lifestyle Factors

Curtail or Eliminate Napping

The effects of napping have been well studied. With healthy sleepers, short naps (<30 minutes) can be beneficial with increased wakefulness and performance, while naps greater than 90 minutes are likely to disrupt nighttime sleep.[125] Too much napping can reduce one's sleep drive and decrease the pressure to sleep at night.

Decrease Time in Bed

As we'll soon discover in subsequent chapters, spending too much time in bed can negatively influence sleep. It has been found that more time spent in bed can lead to sleep that is shallower and fragmented. The recommendation is to reduce time spent in bed to slightly less than before sleep problems developed.[125]

Keep Regular Sleep Times

Regular sleep times can be helpful to maintain consistency with a person's circadian clock which is important in regulating one's sleep.

Exercise Regularly

Exercise, a foundation of any health care provider's toolkit, has been found to help improve sleep. It appears that exercise helps sleep by increasing one's core body temperature and the resulting compensatory drop in body temperature.

The timing of exercise seems to have an impact on the quality of one's sleep. Exercise early in the morning doesn't seem to have an impact on sleep that night, but exercise in the early evening can have a benefit. Hauri recommends that those with sleep difficulties exercise aerobically more than 3 times a week starting 4-6 hours before bedtime.

It seems that the benefit of exercise centers around the increased temperature during exercise and the resulting rebound cooling that takes place following exercise. This may explain why some people find it easier to fall asleep after a hot bath.[125]

Limit or Avoid Caffeine

Caffeine is known to negatively impact sleep. Caffeine's effect on sleep is thought to come primarily through its blocking effect of adenosine receptors. Adenosine is believed to be a sleep promoting substance helping to increase the sleep drive. Caffeine blocks the build-up of this sleep drive.[128] Interestingly, the half-life of caffeine appears to increase with age and its effects are longer lasting in older adults.[130]

Each person has a different level of sensitivity to caffeine. For some people, they may tolerate caffeinated beverages in the morning, while others may need to avoid caffeine altogether.

It is generally recommended to avoid caffeine containing beverages in the afternoon and evening and limiting intake to one cup in the morning. A study of healthy individuals discovered that taking caffeine up to six hours before bedtime still impacted subjective and objective sleep measurements.[130] Unfortunately, the amount of caffeine was equivalent to four cups of coffee which likely doesn't parallel typical behavior.

Hauri points out that some people who are regular coffee drinkers sleep better when they have caffeine before bed. This may be due to the disruptive effects of caffeine withdrawal which may prevent sleep from occurring.[125]

Avoid Smoking

Nicotine is a stimulant and promotes wakefulness and arousal. Nicotine has been shown to:

- Increase difficulties in falling asleep
- Decrease total sleep time

- Increase frequency of early morning awakenings
- Decrease REM
- Decrease slow wave sleep[130]

Avoid Alcohol

The evidence of alcohol on sleep is well documented. Taking alcohol near bedtime does make it easier to fall asleep with increased SWS earlier in the night. Unfortunately, as the night progresses, sleep becomes shallower with more arousals. There has been some research showing that sleep is negatively impacted even when consumed six hours before bedtime.[130]

Eat a Light Snack Before Bed

A light snack can help to minimize the impact of hunger on sleep. However, those with gastroesophageal reflux disease (GERD) should avoid eating before bed.[125]

Limit all liquids before bedtime

Those who frequently get up at night may find limiting liquid intake before bed helpful.

Attitudes and Thoughts

Avoid Trying Hard to Sleep

Frustration with being unable to sleep can increase one's state of arousal and decrease the ability to sleep. Some people find it helpful watching TV or reading to reduce their anxiety / frustration with falling asleep.[125]

Relaxing activities before sleep

Unwinding before bed can help to reduce hyperarousal and prepare the mind and body for rest.

Make a Worry List

As Hauri has noted, people with sleep difficulties can often sabotage their sleep with racing thoughts, preventing sleep from occurring. His recommendation for patients with this difficulty was the following:

- In the early evening, spend 20 minutes making a list of your worries or concerns.
- Review these concerns and identify one small action that you could take tomorrow to help with this concern.
- Next, write down your course of action that will be taken the next day.

Key Take-Aways

There are a few key take-aways regarding sleep hygiene:

- Sleep hygiene rules shouldn't be followed blindly but should be tailored and nuanced to the needs of each patient.
- Sleep hygiene is typically not enough to change people with chronic insomnia.

Technology Use

Although not specifically identified in the sleep hygiene literature, the use of technology is an important sleep hygiene consideration.

Recent research shows the negative impact that mobile devices and screen time have on sleep. In a 2016 study, increased screen time was correlated with decreased sleep quality, decreased sleep duration, decreased sleep efficiency and increased sleep onset latency.[131]

EXERCISE

Exercise has been found helpful to improve sleep quality.

As health care providers, we understand the power of exercise to improve quality of life.

With regards to sleep, evidence supports a positive relationship between sleep and exercise and the relationship appears to be directional in nature. There is evidence to show that increased sleep improves physical activity in older adults.[132,133] Conversely, research generally shows the power of exercise to improve sleep. However, this relationship is somewhat less established.

On the whole, the majority of studies reviewed showed the positive impact of exercise on sleep. For example, in a study by Yang et al, exercise training programs in adults over the age of 40 resulted in:

- Improved sleep quality
- Decreased sleep latency
- Decreased use of sleep medications[134]

Another supportive study showed that 12 months of regular exercise in the morning or early afternoon was more effective than health education in patients with moderate chronic sleep problems.[117]

Physical activity improved a wide range of sleep indicators in a study with adults with chronic insomnia. Improvements were seen in: sleep quality, sleep latency, sleep duration, sleep efficiency and daytime dysfunction.[135]

The 16 week program consisted of four exercise sessions per week with the following parameters:

Conditioning period (Initial 4-6 Weeks):

Week 1: 10-15 minutes/ day at 55% max HR as measured with a heart rate monitor

Week 2: 15-20 minutes/ day at 60% max HR

Week 3: 20-25 minutes/ day at 65% max HR

Week 4: 25-30 minutes/ day at 70% Max HR

Week 5 - 6: up to 75% of max HR for 30-40 minutes

Post Conditioning Period (Remainder of the Program):

Weeks 7-16: 4x/week: Two 20-minute sessions or one 30-40 minute session at 75% Max HR, of at least two of: walking, stationary bicycle or treadmill.

Exercise in Older Adults

However, there appears to be some conflicting results with respect to the effect of exercise on sleep in older adults. While one study showed that sedentary behaviors resulted in decreased sleep efficiency in older adults, another study found that exercise training had no significant effect on sleep characteristics in healthy, older adults.[136,137]

In one particular study involving the elderly, participants engaged in a 10-week high intensity progressive resistance training program of large muscle groups (including chest press, overhead pulldown, leg press, knee flexion) at 80% one rep max intensity for 3 days a week, with sessions lasting 1 hour with 5 minutes of stretching.[10]

The result? An improvement in both short and long term subjective sleep quality, specifically a 35% improvement in mean PSQI.

In a study with older women who participated in walking or dancing as part of a community program for at least 60 minutes, four times per week, researchers found:

- Total sleep time (TST) was higher
- Mean wake up after sleep onset (WASO) was lower
- Perception of sleep quality was higher[138]

Exercise and Sleep Apnea

In a study which involved subjects with moderate-to-severe sleep apnea syndrome, positive results were also seen. Subjects completed two exercise sessions per week, specifically:

- 1x weekly 2 hour aerobic exercise (jogging, games, gymnastics)
- 1x weekly 2 hour power exercise (repetitive light weight lifting) for a period of six months.

No adverse outcomes were reported. Improvements were noted in subjects' respiratory disturbance index (RDI) and no change to their BMI or body weight was noted. However, no change in sleep architecture was observed during this study.[139]

MIND-BODY THERAPIES

There is evidence to support the use of mindfulness-based meditation in insomnia.

Overview

Given our understanding of the impact of cognition and arousal on insomnia, it stands to reason that mind-body therapies may be of benefit in those suffering with insomnia. Relaxation, meditation and other mind-body therapies are used extensively by people suffering from insomnia.[140] Although not recent, a 2002 survey revealed that nearly 20% used complementary and alternative medicine (CAM) to treat their insomnia.[141] A study in 2007 showed that 45% of adults with insomnia had used at least one form of CAM therapy in the past year.[142] One can imagine that these numbers have continued this upward trend since these studies.

Although used extensively by patients, it is important to understand the evidence for these therapies and their ability to influence insomnia outcomes.

Relaxation

Relaxation helps promote sleep as it reduces anxiety and muscle tension, as well as supports a calm mind. Common forms of relaxation are imaging-guided relaxation, transcendental meditation and progressive muscle relaxation (PMR).

In a systematic review of alternative sleep therapies, a total of 25 relaxation intervention studies were included. Unfortunately, the majority were negative and report that results were inconclusive. Of the studies looking at relaxation for those experiencing sleep problems, nearly 40% reported negative results. Although relaxation can be a useful technique for personal peace and calm, it does not look to provide a convincing effect on those struggling with disrupted sleep.[140]

Mindfulness-based Meditation

Mindfulness-based meditation has increasingly become a popular form of meditation and was popularized by Jon Kabat-Zinn in the 1990s. Mindfulness is drawing one's awareness to the present moment with an attitude of acceptance.[143]

Mindfulness-based meditation is both accessible and low cost. In a study comparing the effects of meditation versus sleep hygiene, researchers demonstrated immediate (post-intervention) improved sleep quality in the mindfulness meditation group compared to the sleep hygiene group. Insomnia and depression symptoms along with fatigue improved, while no differences were noted with anxiety or stress. Unfortunately, no long-term conclusions could be made from the study.[144]

In another study, two meditation-based interventions were evaluated compared to controls (self-monitoring using a sleep diary). Researchers evaluated both mindfulness-based stress reduction (MBSR) and mindfulness-based therapy for insomnia (MBTI) (which combines mindfulness with CBT-I). The results of the study showed significantly reduced total wake time and pre-sleep arousal levels immediately and at 6 months in both the MBSR and MBTI groups. There were no significant differences between both groups immediately post treatment, but the MBTI group had a lower insomnia severity index (ISI) at 6 months.[145]

There appears to be some promise in offering mindfulness meditation programs using the internet as a delivery mechanism. A self-report-based study by Boettcher et al demonstrated that this stand-alone and unguided treatment helped to decrease anxiety, depression and insomnia, with results maintained for anxiety and insomnia at 6 months, while depressive symptoms returned.[146]

In another study, cognitive behavioral therapy for insomnia (CBT-I) was shown to have the upper hand compared to MBSR. Researchers evaluated cancer patients with insomnia and found that CBT-I had better outcomes in subjective sleep onset latency (SOL), sleep efficiency, quality and dysfunctional sleep beliefs. However, both groups showed significant improvements in outcomes for wake after sleep onset (WASO), total sleep time (TST), stress and mood disturbance.[147]

Research shows promise with incorporating mindfulness based meditation into a CBT-I program. It does appear that further research is needed to evaluate the impact of meditation on populations such as the elderly and those with chronic pain conditions.

Tai Chi and Yoga

Movement based systems such as tai chi and yoga have also shown positive effects with regards to sleep. In a systematic review of mind-body interventions on sleep quality, the investigators evaluated 31 studies evaluating mind-body movement therapies including tai chi, yoga and qi gong. More than half of the studies showed positive immediate effects, and a subset of studies incorporating sleep measures showed yoga to have the highest amount of positive evidence. The authors conclude that there is some positive evidence for these therapies especially in certain patient populations (e.g. elderly, cancer patients).[140]

To help evaluate mind-body therapies, research investigators evaluated tai chi compared to an active control group receiving health education in patients with moderate sleep disturbances. They found that tai chi attained a treatment response for poor sleep quality that comparable to other behavioral interventions and the magnitude of change was similar to that of pharmacological interventions.[148]

Yoga's popularity continues to increase and studies do support the benefit of yoga on sleep. There are a number of studies showing subjective improvements with sleep from practicing yoga. Other studies have shown that sleep quality, efficiency, duration and latency have improved with yoga.[149] A systematic review on yoga's influence on sleep in older adults has shown that yoga improved sleep quality by decreasing anxiety through reducing sympathetic activity and psychophysiological arousal.[150]

OTHER THERAPIES

Acupuncture appears to show some benefit to improve sleep, but evidence is limited.

Manual Therapy

It was difficult to find any studies looking at the effect of manual therapy on sleep. However, I did find one!

A study by Castro-Sanchez et al, of 89 women and men with fibromyalgia, evaluated the short-term effects of a specific manual therapy protocol on various variables including sleep quality. Sleep quality as measured by the PSQI improved for both male and female subjects in the treatment group at the completion of the intervention (5 weeks).

The intervention involved a once weekly 45-minute session for five weeks and included the following:

- Suboccipital release

- Release of the pectoral region
- Diaphragm release
- Lumbosacral decompression
- Psoas fascia release
- Thoracic spine extension manipulation (in prone)[72]

Acupuncture

A systematic review by Shergis et al, showed a statistically significant improvement with acupuncture over placebo and pharmacotherapy, although they acknowledged evidence is limited due to bias in the studies and heterogeneity.[151]

The review looked at studies where at least one of the insomnia points were used:

- HT 7
- GV 20
- SP 6

Acupuncture is reported to work for insomnia treatment due to acupuncture's interaction with one of sleep's main neurotransmitters: GABA. GABA has an inhibitory effect on the brain and increasing GABA will suppress the central nervous system (CNS). By acting on this pathway, it is performing a similar function as sleep medications such as benzodiazepine and non-benzodiazepine hypnotics.[151]

Various studies have shown the impact on GABA:

- Mice stimulated at HT 7, showed effect on GABA pathways
- Acupuncture of the head showed increase GABA in multiple areas of the brain

- A small study of 48 people, where HT 7 and SP 6 were stimulated, showed increased amount of GABA in cerebrospinal fluid compared to alprazolam

Acupuncture also has been shown to increase melatonin levels, which we know is involved in regulating sleep. Acupuncture has been shown to improve subjective sleep quality and PSQI improvement when compared to sham control (seen with electroacupuncture and acupressure as well). Increased benefit was seen when ear acupressure was added to acupuncture.[151]

SUPPLEMENTS

There is limited evidence for the use of supplements in supporting sleep health.

The use of over-the-counter supplements are popular with people experiencing insomnia. As health professionals, it's important to understand the research and evidence for these biologic compounds. Again, it is important to recognize your professional limitations regarding scope of practice. For healthcare providers such as physiotherapists where it is beyond our scope to provide recommendations regarding medications and supplements, the following is for informational purposes only.

Melatonin

Melatonin is a neurohormone produced by the pineal gland and an important factor in regulating the sleep-wake cycle. Melatonin supplements are a popular sleep remedy and supplements are chemically synthesized or extracted from animal pineal glands.[149] This hormone also tends to decrease with age. As well, beta-blockers and conditions such as chronic pain, myocardial interactions and stroke are associated with decreased levels.

Juarascio et al summarized a number of key melatonin studies and highlighted mixed findings, ranging from reduced sleep latency, improved sleep efficiency, to worsened mood or no effect. A meta-analysis of studies found that there was a significant decrease in sleep onset latency in those with delayed sleep phase syndrome and a small, but significant decrease in sleep onset latency for those with primary insomnia. No change in sleep efficiency or wakefulness after sleep onset were noted. This led the authors to conclude that melatonin's effect was circadian in nature, not sedative.[152]

It appears that short term use (<3 months) is safe and side effects are rare, although higher doses can have daytime side effects such as decreased alertness, headache, dizziness and irritability.[149,152]

However, consideration should be given to certain patient populations:

- Conflicting information regarding the potential of melatonin to have a pro-inflammatory effect in those with autoimmune arthritis

- Potentially help increase the apnea-hypopnea index (AHI) for patients with obstructive sleep apnea (OSA)

- Potential decrease in endogenous melatonin levels in those with bipolar disorder with long-term use (e.g. > 3 months)[152]

Bottom Line: Melatonin primarily benefits circadian rhythm disorders (e.g. delayed sleep phase disorder). It appears that the effect is minimal or non-existent for those suffering from insomnia.

Valerian

Valerian has been used for centuries as a sleep aid and is one of the most common herbal remedies for insomnia. The challenge with valerian is there are over 400 hundred compounds found within the most commonly used valerian species and the active substances continue to remain unknown.[153,] [154] The specific mechanism of action is still unknown. It is thought that valerian impacts specific neurotransmitters such as GABA, adenosine and serotonin.

Given the challenge of identifying the active ingredients within valerian, the evidence for valerian is limited. Placebo controlled studies show no therapeutic benefit of valerian.[154]

Valerian appears to result in decreased time to fall asleep (sleep latency), improved sleep quality and decreased awakenings. It also appears to lengthen stage 3 (N3) sleep.[154]

Sleep architecture, specifically REM sleep, has been found to change in human studies. REM sleep decreases during the early part of the night while increasing later at night. Research suggests a subjective improvement in sleep quality, night awakenings and possibly sleep onset latency.[152] Modest doses of valerian seem to deliver sleep-inducing effects without impacting sleep architecture.

Valerian does appear safe to use and there have been few reported side effects.[153] In terms of safety, it appears that use of valerian for four to six weeks is safe with doses not exceeding 400mg to 900mg of an extract. There appear to be some interaction effects with sedative drugs such as barbiturates and authors urge caution when combining valerian with sedative medications.[152]

L-Tryptophan

L-Tryptophan is an essential amino acid found in food and is used as a sleep aid in many countries. Studies have shown a benefit in decreased nocturnal awakenings along with moderate reductions in sleep latency and is considered of benefit for short-term use (less than four weeks).[50]

5-HTP

5-HTP (5 Hydroxytryptophan) is a naturally occurring amino acid and a precursor to serotonin (neurotransmitter). It is marketed as a sleep aid, but also used for depression and appetite suppression. Small studies appear to improve subjective and objective sleep measures however, studies have been small in number and have methodological limitations. The side effects and drug interactions are not known as 5-HTP has not been well studied in clinical settings.[152]

St. John's Wort

St. John's Wort is a flowering herb and is primarily used for depression, as well as insomnia. It appears that there are typically a number of other substances included in St. John's Wort. The main active ingredients appear to be hypercin and hyperforin. It is suggested that hyperforin inhibits the re-uptake of various neurotransmitters such as serotonin, GABA, dopamine, norepinephrine and L-glutamate.

Studies relating to St. John's Wort and its effect on insomnia are limited. Small sample sizes, the use of healthy subjects with no insomnia and the variations in supplement preparation make it difficult to make any conclusions as to its use and efficacy in insomnia.[152]

Chamomile

Chamomile is another popular remedy for insomnia. It is believed that the sedative effects of chamomile are a result of the benzodiazepine-like compound found in the chamomile flower. Unfortunately, no randomized clinical trials have been done. Animal trials support its role as a mild sedative and anxiolytic. Chamomile may interact with anticoagulant and antiplatelet drugs as well as sedatives (e.g. benzodiazepines).[152]

Hops

Hops, while used primarily in beer, have also been used to treat insomnia, anxiety and tension. It appears that preparations vary widely (with over 100 compounds in hops), making it difficult to isolate the active compounds. Again, research is limited and studies completed have often used hops in combination with other compounds (e.g. valerian). Hops may cause a hyper-sensitivity reaction such as dermatitis, and in reading about this, sleep researchers encouraged caution when taking other CNS depressants or antipsychotics.[152]

Key Take-Aways

- Sleep medication has a role in the treatment of insomnia, but it's important to understand that medication does not cure insomnia.

- There are certain patient populations where CBT-I, the standard of treatment for insomnia, is not of benefit and medications are necessary.

- Sleep hygiene helps set the foundation for healthy sleep but is not enough for those suffering from chronic insomnia.

- Exercise has a positive effect on sleep.

- Research supports incorporating mindfulness practice into a CBT-I program.

- Although a popular insomnia supplement, it appears that melatonin primarily benefits circadian rhythm disorders, not insomnia.

- There are a variety of other natural supplements purported to promote healthy sleep, but research is limited.

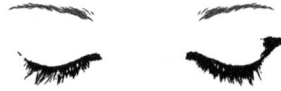

CHAPTER 8

COGNITIVE BEHAVIORAL THERAPY FOR INSOMNIA

Understand the safe and evidence based treatment approach for insomnia.

COVERED IN THIS CHAPTER:

CBT-I Overview

Behavioral Therapies

Cognitive Retraining

CBT-I OVERVIEW

CBT-I is an effective, well-researched treatment framework for those struggling with insomnia.

Defining CBT-I

Cognitive behavioral therapy for insomnia (CBT-I) is a non-pharmacological treatment approach that targets psychological, behavioral and cognitive factors that are perpetuating or exacerbating disrupted sleep.[127] CBT-I is specific training to help patients recognize the relationship between cognition, effect and sleep behavior.

The components of CBT-I include education and instruction in the areas of cognitive therapy, stimulus control, sleep restriction, sleep hygiene and relaxation. The following table provides further details[121]:

Component	Description
Cognitive Therapy	Challenge and replace dysfunctional beliefs and attitudes about sleep and insomnia.
Stimulus Control	Behavioral rules aimed at improving the association of bed and sleep and removing association with stimulating activities.
Sleep Restriction	Behavioral changes limiting time in bed to better match actual sleep duration with the goal of improving sleep drive. The goal is sleep efficiency of >85%.
Sleep Hygiene	Recommendations for environmental factors and habits to support sound sleep (e.g. alcohol, caffeine, napping, etc.).
Relaxation	Techniques found helpful by the patient to reduce cognitive arousal and muscle tension.

Note: Adapted from Trauer et al.

The Research for CBT-I

CBT for insomnia has strong research support. In a systematic review and meta-analysis, researchers Trauer et al determined that CBT-I is an effective treatment for non-comorbid insomnia (not relating to another condition), leading to improved sleep diary outcomes, and should be the initial treatment for insomnia. Their research showed that outcomes from CBT-I were maintained in both early and late follow-up of patients.[121]

In another meta-analysis, researchers determined CBT-I was at least as effective for treating insomnia compared to sleep medications.[123] The limitation of this review, however, was that there were few studies comparing CBT-I to medications.

CBT-I has been shown to benefit 70-80% of those suffering with chronic insomnia and approximately half will experience clinical remission.[127] Of those, one third may even become good sleepers.[4] In a randomized control study by Jacobs et al, results showed that cognitive behavioral therapy (CBT) alone produced long-term benefits in insomnia patients compared to medications or a combination of medications and CBT.[129]

As previously mentioned, the American Academy of Sleep Medicine (AASM) recommends that the first line of treatment for those with chronic insomnia should be CBT-I.[7]

Advantages and Disadvantages

A primary advantage of CBT-I is the lack of medications which come with their own side-effects. CBT-I focuses on addressing the underlying causes perpetuating one's insomnia, and the durable effects noted with CBT-I reduces or eliminates the need for long term medication use. As well, gains can be made relatively quickly (e.g. 6-8 weeks).[123]

Studies also show that older adults can benefit as much as younger and middle-aged adults, but outcomes can be mitigated by the presence of comorbid medical or psychiatric conditions.[155]

However, patients should expect greater daytime sleepiness as there is a reduction in total sleep time during the first few weeks of treatment. Improvements from CBT-I may take 3-4 weeks to occur as the body adjusts.[123]

CBT-I and Non-Sleep Specialists

The research shows strong support for the implementation for CBT for insomnia. The challenge though is the lack of qualified sleep specialists who can administer CBT for insomnia in a wide variety of clinical settings.

Sleep researchers Manber et al set out to evaluate the potential for non-sleep specialists (i.e. mental health providers) to offer CBT-I to their patients. They note that sleep science is not well covered (if covered at all) in many mental health professional programs.[156]

Their initial pilot cohort resulted in positive feedback and a further roll-out of their program protocol was planned.

Sleep researcher Colin Espie puts forward the argument that CBT-I should be delivered in a "stepped care" model to improve delivery and access to CBT-I. This model argues that given CBT-I's flexibility, it can be delivered at varying levels of sophistication and involvement of specialized providers. This stepped model supports the notion of health care clinicians providing CBT-I care for patients and referring to sleep specialists as needed.[157]

Non-Traditional Delivery

More and more, the internet is changing the delivery mechanism of information and health care. Increasingly, internet-based CBT-I programs have been introduced to improve access to their intervention.

A systematic review and meta-analysis of (15 and 13 studies respectively) reported that Internet-delivered CBT-I showed clinically significant improvements in:

- Insomnia severity
- Sleep efficiency (SE)
- Total sleep time (TST)
- Sleep onset latency (SOL)
- Wake time after sleep onset (WASO)

Insomnia improvements were found to remain even over a long follow-up period (e.g. 48 weeks).[158]

BEHAVIORAL THERAPIES

There are a variety of different behavioral strategies that can help to improve the sleep cycle and can be tailored to individual patients.

Stimulus Control

Stimulus control is considered one of the most effective behavior interventions and a core element in CBT-I. The goal of stimulus control is to pair rapid sleep onset with the bedroom. For good sleepers, the bedroom triggers positive associations with sleep through both pre-sleep rituals and environmental cues. The opposite is true for poor sleepers.[4,159] For the poor sleeper, the bedroom unfortunately becomes paired with staying awake.

For those suffering with insomnia, the bed has become a cue for arousal, which prevents sleep. Poor sleepers have spent hours and hours of wakefulness in bed, often frustrated, angered and worried about their lack of sleep. This increased psychological arousal makes it impossible for sleep to occur and instead arousal is conditioned to occur with the bedroom. The rules set out in stimulus control treatment are meant to reshape this conditioned arousal and improve the circadian rhythm and sleep drive.[30]

There are five steps associated with stimulus control (adapted from Espie & Kyle) which are:

- Go to bed only when sleepy.
- Use your bed only for sleeping (and sex). All other activities such as reading, watching TV and eating are prohibited.
- Get out of bed if you're unable to sleep after 15 minutes. Leave the bedroom and go to another room until you feel sleepy again. This process should be repeated as many times as necessary during the night.
- Set up an alarm clock for consistent rising time each morning.
- Avoid all daytime napping.[159]

Manber & Carney provide some specific recommendations and clarification regarding sleep restriction rules. First off, it's important to distinguish sleepiness vs tiredness. As they suggest, sleepiness is "being on the verge of dozing off and almost having to struggle to stay awake" while fatigue/tiredness is "having low energy and low motivation to stay awake."[31]

It is important to make note that activities to engage in if unable to sleep should be calming and not arousing. For example, watching a suspenseful TV show would increase psychological arousal which would prevent the body from being sleep ready. Manber & Carney also state that activities that are too engaging or arousing will mask sleepiness. Individual preference and tolerance must also be taken into account, as a calming activity for one person may not be for another. It can be helpful to develop a list of calming activities to discuss with patients.

It is important to understand that changes to bed-sleep pairing will take longer than one night. As Manber & Carney highlight, patients can be worried that they will need to stay up all night because of a lack of sleepiness. It is important for patients to understand that this retraining should focus on the long-term goal even though there may initially be some bumps along the way.

As well, it can be a challenge to get out of bed at the same time each day and even though an alarm may sound, people may still stay in bed. It's important to get out of bed within 10-15 minutes of waking in the morning. This will strengthen the circadian rhythm. As Manber & Carney highlight, having varying sleep wake times creates a form of "behavioral jet lag."

There will be situations where a patient may have difficulty getting out of bed due to limited mobility or pain. An alternative strategy called counter control has been found to be nearly as effective as the sleep restriction protocol.[31]

With this strategy, the patient can sit in bed and enjoy calm activities such as light reading, TV watching, listening to a podcast, etc. Although it appears counter-productive at first glance, the premise is based on the concept that these bed activities reduces one's focus on trying to sleep as well as the frustration of not sleeping. This distraction aims to lower the arousal state so sleep is possible.

Sleep Restriction Therapy

Sleep restriction therapy is another central component to a CBT-I program. The goal of restriction therapy is to consolidate sleep and improve sleep quality by more closely matching sleep time to the time spent in bed. Those suffering from sleep disturbance often spend longer periods in bed in an attempt to increase their sleep time. The increased time in bed with limited sleep results in poor sleep efficiency. This decreased sleep efficiency results in increased sleep fragmentation and less deep sleep.

Sleep restriction therapy focuses on reducing sleep fragmentation as well as improving one's sleep drive so as to improve sleep architecture.

The following list adapted from Espie & Kyle highlight the guidelines for sleep restriction therapy:

- The patient should record their sleep behavior using a sleep diary for a period of two weeks with the goal of getting an average nightly sleep duration (round to nearest 15 minutes).
- The therapist and the patient collaboratively set a morning wake time.
- A bed time is then calculated by subtracting the average sleep time from the agreed upon wake time.
- Patients are instructed to not go to bed before the designated bed time and to not get up later than the agreed upon wake time.
- Follow this schedule every night including weekends.

- Modify this sleep window based on weekly sleep efficiency values. If sleep efficiency is greater than 90%, the sleep window can be increased by 15 minutes. If below 85%, the sleep window decreases by 15 minutes.

- To improve patient compliance, add an additional 30 minutes to the total time a patient can spend in bed.[159]

Manber & Carney provide slightly different sleep efficiency numbers and provide an algorithm for changing time in bed values based on the previous week's sleep diary data:

- **If SE >85%:** increase sleep time by 15 minutes per night. They suggest increasing to 30 minutes if daytime sleepiness is present.

- **If SE is between 80-85%:** Leave the sleep window unaltered or adjust based on the most recent week's sleep numbers.

- **If SE < 80%:** Troubleshoot potential issues relating to patient adherence and recalculate sleep window based on the most recent week.[31]

Various sleep researchers highlight that adjusting one's sleep window can result in acute and mild sleep deprivation.[31, 159] This increased sleep deprivation can help to improve sleep drive and reduce excessive arousal pre-sleep. However, there are some safety considerations. The total time in bed should never be less than 5 hours and if daytime sleepiness is severe, this protocol should not be followed.

A more gentle form of sleep restriction therapy is sleep compression therapy. It focuses on providing a gradual approach to adjusting one's total time in bed rather than the abrupt approach of sleep restriction therapy. In this approach, the total time in bed is subtracted from the total sleep time. If a 6 week program is implemented, 1/6th of the difference between TST and TIB would be reduced on a weekly basis.[31]

A number of authors have highlighted that the term "sleep restriction therapy" can be anxiety producing for patients who already feel that their sleep is restricted. They suggest using alternative terms such as "sleep efficiency training" or "time-in-bed restriction."[31]

COGNITIVE RETRAINING

Addressing poor thinking about sleep is important in improving sleep.

The Role of Cognition

The previously described behavioral strategies are important in resetting the circadian clock, improving sleep drive and improving behavioral conditioning by pairing the bed with sleep. However, those suffering from insomnia typically have thoughts, beliefs and attitudes about sleep that are limiting their ability to sleep well.

Falling asleep is just that. It's a passive, involuntary process where one allows oneself to enter into a sleep state. Good sleepers don't do anything specific to fall asleep, whereas poor sleepers increase their attention and effort to sleep.[160]

Earlier in the book, we talked about a model for insomnia (the predisposing, precipitating and perpetuating (3P) model). There have been additional models proposed to better understand insomnia. One such model attempts to explain ongoing insomnia and the causative role that our thoughts play. This model highlights the increased psychological arousal and stress that results in ongoing insomnia. As previously mentioned, the concept of arousal is important. Low arousal is needed for one to fall asleep. Unfortunately, worry, rumination, hyper-vigilance and tension about sleep all lead to increased autonomic arousal and emotional distress.[161]

This model also explores the challenges with cognition that occur during both the daytime and nighttime in supporting ongoing insomnia. Unfortunately, those who struggle with insomnia have been found to have a harder time managing life and work stress. This sets one up for increased arousal and distress which can carry over into the evening. Additionally, those with insomnia have been found to have excess pre-sleep cognitive activity which tends to be more negative in nature. As well, patients will complain of their frustration with a 'racing mind' and the inability to empty one's mind for sleep.

This can lead to those with insomnia paying increased attention to specific physical and environmental sleep related cues. This can include increased monitoring when trying to fall asleep, as well as being more aware of midday fatigue.

Another challenge that needs to be addressed for those with insomnia is identifying and challenging specific safety behaviors. These are strategies that patients will pursue to avoid a particular sleep related outcome. The challenge is that these safety behaviors tend to confirm inaccurate beliefs. An example of a safety behavior would be a patient worried that they won't be able to fall asleep because they've had a stressful day at work. They may then have a drink to help them relax. They may fall asleep more quickly, but their sleep will be poor. Unfortunately, this person will believe that alcohol helps their sleep even though it has negatively impacted their overall sleep.[161]

There are definite similarities noticed in reviewing this model and the wind-up and sensitization processes that take place with persistent pain. Without challenging the various beliefs and thoughts surrounding a patient's insomnia, it is more difficult to ensure compliance and improvement.

Key Areas of Cognitive Challenge

As Morin et al highlights, there are three key thought areas facing those struggling with insomnia. They are:

- **Unrealistic expectations about sleep**: "I must get 9 hours of uninterrupted sleep every night to function."

- **Faulty causal attributions relating to their insomnia:** "My insomnia comes entirely from my anxious personality."

- **Amplifying the consequences of poor sleep:** "I'm going to bomb my work presentation because I slept poorly." [127]

Another cognitive hurdle is one's beliefs about sleep effort. Those with insomnia believe they need to actively control the sleep process and they fail to recognize the passive nature of sleep.

Cognitive therapy within the context of insomnia treatment focuses on changing specific beliefs, expectations (i.e. cognitions) and cognitive processes around dysfunctional sleep. Cognitive processes include excessive self-monitoring and worrying, which impede healthy sleep. [127]

Manber & Carney outline the components of cognitive therapy treatment:

- Provide relevant information to correct inaccurate thoughts and beliefs about sleep

- Identify, with the patient, the validity and usefulness of thoughts using different techniques such as Socratic questioning, cost-benefit analyses and behavioral experiments

- Help patients replace inaccurate thoughts with more beneficial and accurate thoughts

- Help patients apply insights they gleaned about their sleep thoughts and beliefs to manage poor sleep when it happens[31]

Key Messages in Cognitive Therapy

There are a number of key messages that sleep researcher Charles Morin et al recommend to communicate within cognitive therapy. These messages are highlighted below:

- Have realistic expectations about your sleep requirements and daytime energy.

- Don't blame your insomnia on daytime problems. There may be other reasons that are contributing to your daytime functioning (e.g. conflicts, family worries).

- Don't try to sleep, it will just make things worse.

- Avoid making sleep too important. Even though sleep is important and should be a priority, it shouldn't be the central focus of your life.

- Avoid catastrophizing after a poor night's sleep. Even though insomnia can be unpleasant, it doesn't mean it's dangerous to your health in the short term.

- Build up some tolerance to the effects of insomnia. If you've struggled with insomnia, the likelihood is you'll experience it again, so develop strategies on how to cope after a poor sleep night.[127]

Cognitive Therapy Tools

There are a number of cognitive therapy techniques to use in addressing this roadblock to sleep. They include:

Worry Worksheet

Often, those struggling with insomnia find themselves unable to quiet their minds for sleep and are actively problem-solving life or work challenges during this time of quiet. A simple pre-sleep writing assignment is where patients outline their concern in one column and possible solutions in the next column. This process allows patients to identify and record their worries and then outline possible next, immediate steps that they can take to solve these worries.[127]

Having the patient work through the worries of their day (preferably earlier in the evening) through journaling helps to reduce one's need for processing this information when trying to sleep. Instead, the patient proactively addresses these worries earlier in the day so they are free to fall asleep.

Thought Record

The worry worksheet is a thought record that is a classic cognitive therapy tool for changing negative thinking. The worry worksheet has the following columns:

- Situation
- Mood (Intensity 0-100%)
- Thoughts
- Evidence for this thought
- Evidence against this thought
- Reframed thought

- Feel differently now?[127]

The process of writing out one's thoughts helps to add much needed perspective and provides an opportunity to challenge thoughts previously accepted automatically.

Socratic Questioning

This form of questioning helps patients to become aware of information relevant to the conversation regarding their insomnia but may have been unaware of previously.[31] Questions such as "What do you mean by…" and "What's the implication of…" provide a helpful template in the phrasing of this type of questioning.

Cost-Benefit Analysis

This cognitive therapy technique helps patients evaluate the usefulness of a particular belief relating to their sleep by evaluating the cost and benefit of that belief.[31]

Behavioral Experiments

One of the challenges with insomnia is that patients will engage in strategies to avoid behaviors. This was highlighted in safety behaviors that patients engage in. Behavioral experiments are a strategy for a patient to test a different approach and evaluate the impact. For example, someone who believes that getting up at the same time during the week as during the weekend may test this strategy to see what the impact is on daytime sleepiness by testing both approaches.

Paradoxical Intention

Paradoxical intention is a technique that challenges patients to engage in their most feared behavior.[4] It is recommended for those who have an intense focus on sleep, sleep loss and consequences of sleep loss. It's believed that this approach helps reduce performance anxiety relating to sleep. One example is having the patient try to stay awake. They are encouraged to keep their eyes open, give up any effort to fall asleep and give up any worry about being awake.[159]

Key Take-Aways

- CBT-I is an effective, well-researched treatment framework for those struggling with insomnia.

- There is research supporting the implementation of CBT-I by non-sleep specialists.

- Stimulus control is important to reshape the behavioral conditioning of the bed with wakefulness.

- Restricting one's sleep is an important component of CBT-I and aims to support the build-up of sleep drive to improve overall sleep architecture.

- Certain cognitive beliefs are common among those suffering from insomnia and need to be challenged.

- There are various cognitive therapy tools to support addressing cognitive barriers to healthy sleep.

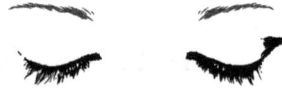

CHAPTER 9

CONCLUSION & NEXT STEPS

Sleep health matters. More than ever our sleep is being challenged with increased work/life demands and our increasingly persistent use of technology.

Writing this book has been a journey. A rewarding one. Sleep medicine is an ever evolving area of research and clinical practice. The treatment options available for those suffering with insomnia are so much more than offering a few basic sleep hygiene recommendations.

I'm more convinced than ever that sleep health is absolutely critical to the lives of our patients. As healthcare providers, I believe we have an important role in helping our patients with sleep.

The study of the relationship between sleep and pain will continue to evolve and I believe the findings will increasingly point to an integrated relationship between sleep and pain.

We owe it to our patients to improve our understanding of sleep and begin to have conversations about this pillar of health.

A CLINICAL TOOLKIT TO SUPPORT YOUR PRACTICE

Reading a book is a good start to knowledge acquisition and translation, but it's only a start. The challenge now is to begin the transformational process of turning information into knowledge. From the outset I wanted to create a set of resources that would not only give information, but help clinicians in their practice.

That's why I created a number of therapist integration and patient education tools beyond this book. I developed these tools to accelerate information-to-practice and help you improve your patients understanding of their sleep health.

The tools I have created support the individual practitioner as well as the clinic.

5 Steps to Start Incorporating Sleep Health into Practice

This easy-to-read 5 page guide gives you my recommended steps to getting started with sleep health in the clinic. These are the steps I wish I had taken when starting out on this journey of sleep health.

Key Sleep Screening Questions Cheat Sheet

It's easy to get overwhelmed with questions to start asking your patients. This simple PDF handout gives you the 4 key questions you should be asking your patients about their sleep and gives you visual cues to actually remember the questions to ask.

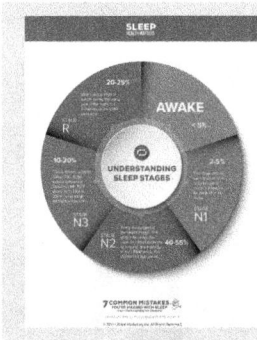

Understanding Sleep Stages Visual

This full color visual can be an excellent support tool to help you educate your patients about the stages of sleep. Supporting key points are included for each stage, so you're cued as to what to share with patients.

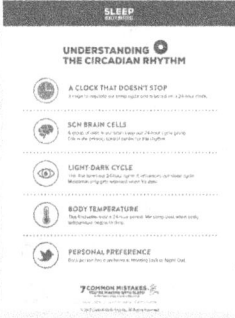

Explain the Basics of the Circadian Rhythm

The circadian rhythm is an important topic to cover with patients. This full color visual is professionally designed and gives you the key points to highlight about the different elements of the circadian rhythm.

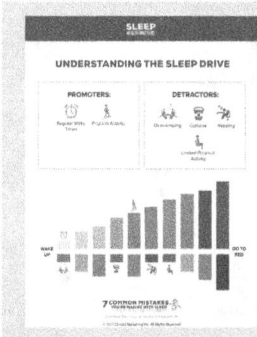

Understanding the Sleep Drive Visual

There are a number of factors that influence the internal drive to sleep. Professionally designed, this graphic highlights the factors that can increase OR decrease the sleep drive and thereby affect sleep efficiency.

An Overview of the Sleep Cycle

Typically the sleep cycle graphs are complicated and hard to understand. We've created a full color visual that is simple to understand and highlights the key takeaways for explaining the sleep cycle.

Screening for Sleep Apnea: The STOP-Bang

The STOP-Bang is a validated obstructive sleep apnea questionnaire that can help to identify those patients who are at a higher risk for sleep apnea. The handout provides a handy weight and BMI chart for easy scoring of the STOP-Bang.

The 4 Key Principles for Healthy Sleep Patient Handout

This one-page color visual highlights the key principles that patients should follow when promoting healthy sleep. This can serve as a great handout for patients.

Clinic Posters to Support Patient Education

Educate your patients about sleep with visual impact. Educate patients about the sleep stages, 4 key questions to self-assess sleep health and key questions to identify risk of sleep apnea. Handouts and high-resolution print-ready PDFs enable you to easily print these posters to a large size (18"x24") and display in your clinical environment.

NEXT STEPS

To learn more about the clinician toolkits, please visit www.sleephealthmatters.com/packages

SLEEP HEALTH RESOURCES

OUTCOME MEASURES

Consensus Sleep Diary

This is an excellent sleep diary that also provides detailed instructions for each element of the sleep diary. This external link provides a printable PDF that can be filled out by the patient in the morning.

[http://bit.ly/consensussleepdiary]

PSQI

The PSQI is the most popular sleep outcome measure and provides a global sleep quality score. The outcome measure also provides insight into various sleep components including: subjective sleep quality, sleep latency, sleep duration, sleep efficiency, sleep disturbances, daytime function and sleeping medication. This external link provides a printable PDF that can be completed by the patient.

[http://bit.ly/psqi-measure]

DBAS 16

This is a shortened version of the original DBAS which highlights non-supportive beliefs about sleep. The external link provides a printable PDF that can be completed by the patient. **[http://bit.ly/dbas16]**

Epworth Sleepiness Scale

This scale provides a short questionnaire relating to issues of daytime sleepiness. This external link provides a printable PDF that can be completed by the patient. **[http://bit.ly/ess-measure]**

SLEEP SPECIALIST REFERRALS

Sleep Clinic Map (Canada)

This website allows you to search for sleep clinics across Canada and filter by the following categories: • Dental Sleep Medicine Providers • Insomnia Treatment Providers • Sleep Clinics

[http://bit.ly/sleepclinics-canada]

CBT-I PATIENT RESOURCES

Constructive Worry Worksheet

This worksheet can help to reduce patient anxieties while preparing for sleep and is recommended to be completed in the early evening. The link provides a printable PDF with instructions and the worry worksheet that can be completed by the patient.

[http://bit.ly/constructiveworry]

Overcoming Insomnia Workbook

This is a workbook developed by sleep researchers Edinger & Carney that provides basic education regarding sleep health and CBT-I. It is nicely laid out and easy for a patient to read and complete. Basic troubleshooting recommendations are provided such as difficulties avoiding napping. However, there are no specific recommendations regarding patients dealing with chronic pain, etc.

[http://bit.ly/overcominginsomniaworkbook]

INTERNET-BASED CBT-I PROGRAMS

Sleepio

Sleepio is an online CBT-I program for patients. It is a paid website program which costs $300 USD per year. Health professionals have their own portal access where they can see patient progress.

[https://www.sleepio.com]

My Shuti

My Shuti is an online CBT-I program for patients. It costs $135 for 16 weeks of access. They have a professional program which costs a little more, but gives a window into a patient's progress for health professionals.

[http://www.myshuti.com]

Go! To Sleep

This is a 6 week online CBT-I program delivered by the Cleveland Clinic of Wellness. The cost for the program is $40 USD.

[http://bit.ly/gotosleepapp]

Restore CBT-I

This is a 5-week CBT-I program that can be completed online. Pricing is in British pounds and costs £99.

[http://bit.ly/restorecbti]

GUIDED RELAXATION APPS

Stop, Breathe & Think

This is a great iPhone/Android app that offers a variety of guided breathing exercises. For a complete review of the app, read the blog post published on ignitephysio.

[https://www.stopbreathethink.com]

Meditation Oasis

Meditation Oasis provides a number of different relaxation and meditation apps. Reviews on iTunes are positive.

[http://bit.ly/meditationoasis]

Headspace

This meditation website (and accompanying mobile app) was started by a Buddhist monk and offers a free basic package and a subscription plan for additional meditations and instruction.

[http://www.headspace.com]

TECHNOLOGY SUPPORT

F.lux

For those who use a Mac computer, you'll enjoy this program that adjusts screen brightness based on time of day. The intensity of the screen light is adjusted to help reduce excess light triggering that can impact one's circadian rhythm.

[https://justgetflux.com]

Sleep Cycle App

This is a free app from the Apple App Store that will measure your sleep cycle simply by having your phone beside your bed stand.

[https://www.sleepcycle.com]

REFERENCES

1. Colten, H. & Altevogt, B. (2006). Sleep disorders and sleep deprivation: An unmet public health problem. Washington, DC: The National Academies Press.

2. Bentley, A. (2007). Pain perception during sleep and circadian influences: The experimental evidence. In G. Lavigne, B. J. Sessle, M. Choiniere, & P. J. Soja (Eds.), Sleep and pain (pp. 235-266). Seattle, WA: IASP Press.

3. Lockley, S. & Foster R. (2012). Sleep: A very short introduction. London: Oxford University Press.

4. Morin, C., Hauri, P., Espie, C., Spielman, A., Buyssee, D. & Bootzin, R. (1999). Nonpharmacologic treatment of chronic insomnia. SLEEP, 22(8),1134-1156.

5. Morin, C., Hauri, P., Espie, C., Spielman, A., Buyssee, D. & Bootzin, R. (1999). Nonpharmacologic treatment of chronic insomnia. SLEEP, 22(8),1134-1156.

6. Malow, B. (2016). Approach to the patient with disordered sleep. In M. Kryger, T. Roth & W. Dement (Eds.), Principles and practice of sleep medicine (6th ed., pp. 573-575). St. Louis, MO: Elsevier

7. Sateia, M. J., Buysse, D. J., Krystal, A. D., Neubauer, D. N., & Heald, J. L. (2017). Clinical Practice Guideline for the Pharmacologic Treatment of Chronic Insomnia in Adults: An American Academy of Sleep Medicine Clinical Practice Guideline. Journal of Clinical Sleep Medicine, 13(02), 307–349.

8. Lichstein, K. L., Taylor, D., McCrae, C. & Ruiter, M. (2016). Insomnia: Epidemiology and risk factors. In M. Kryger, T. Roth & W. Dement (Eds.), Principles and practice of sleep medicine (6th ed., pp. 761-768). St. Louis, MO: Elsevier Saunders.

9. Llanas, A. C., Hachul, H., Bittencourt, L. R., & Tufik, S. (2008). Physical therapy reduces insomnia symptoms in postmenopausal women. Maturitas, 61(3), 281-284.

10. Singh, N., Clements, K. & Fiatarone, M. (1997). Sleep, sleep deprivation, and daytime activities: A randomized controlled trial of the effect of exercise on sleep. SLEEP, 20(2), 95-101.

11. Archbold, K. (2011). Pediatric sleep disorders. In N. Redeker & G. McEnany (Eds.), Sleep disorders and sleep promotion in nursing practice (pp. 219-232). New York, NY: Springer.

12. Buxton, O., Broussard, J., Zahl, A. & Hall, M. (2014). Effects of sleep deficiency on hormones, cytokines and metabolism. In S. Redline & N.A. Berger (Eds.), Impact of sleep and sleep disturbances on obesity and cancer (pp. 25-50). New York, NY: Springer.

13. Orzel-Gryglewska, J. (2010). Consequences of sleep deprivation. International Journal of Occupational Medicine and Environmental Health. 23(1), 95-114.

14. Coren, S. (2009). Sleep health and its assessment and management in physical therapy practice: The evidence. Physiotherapy Theory and Practice, 25(5-6), 442-452.

15. Shneerson, J. M. (2000). Handbook of sleep medicine. Malden, MA: Blackwell Science.

16. AlDabal, L. & BaHammam, A. S. (2011). Metabolic, endocrine, and immune consequences of sleep deprivation. The Open Respiratory Medicine Journal, 5(1), 31-43

17. Valenza, M. C., Rodenstein, D. O., & Fernández-de-las-Peñas, C. (2011). Consideration of sleep dysfunction in rehabilitation. Journal of Bodywork and Movement Therapies, 15(3), 262-267.

18. Delaney, L. J. (2016). The role of sleep in patient recovery. Australian Nursing & Midwifery Journal, 23(7), 26–29.

19. Simpson, N., & Dinges, D. F. (2007). Sleep and Inflammation. Nutrition Reviews, 65(12), 244–252.

20. Vgontzas, A. N., Papanicolaou, D. A., Bixler, E. O., Lotsikas, A., Zachman, K., Kales, A., ... & Hermida, R. C. (1999). Circadian interleukin-6 secretion and quantity and depth of sleep. The Journal of Clinical Endocrinology & Metabolism, 84(8), 2603-2607.

21. Opp, M.R. (2005). Cytokines and sleep. Sleep Medicine Reviews, 9(5), 355-364.

22. Dinges, D. F., Douglas, S. D., Zaugg, L., Campbell, D. E., McMann, J. M., Whitehouse, W. G., ... & Orne, M. T. (1994). Leukocytosis and natural killer cell function parallel neurobehavioral fatigue induced by 64 hours of sleep deprivation. The Journal of Clinical Investigation, 93(5), 1930-1939.

23. National Sleep Foundation (2017). What is Insomnia? Retrieved from http://sleepdisorders.sleepfoundation.org/chapter-2-insomnia/what-is-insomnia/on13 March 2018

24. Morin, C. Belanger, L., LeBlank, M., Ivers, H, et al (2009). The natural history of insomnia: A population-based 3-year longitudinal study. Archives of Internal Medicine. 169(5),447-453.

25. Buysse, D. J. (2013). Insomnia. JAMA 309(7), 706-716.

26. Lichstein, K. L., Durrence, H. H., Taylor, D. J., Bush, A. J., & Riedel, B. W. (2003). Quantitative criteria for insomnia. Behaviour Research and Therapy, 41(4), 427-445.

27. Roth, T. (2007). Insomnia: definition, prevalence, etiology, and consequences. Journal of Clinical Sleep Medicine, 3(5 Suppl), S7–10.

28. Reite, M., Weissberg, M., Ruddy, J. (2009). Clinical manual for evaluation and treatment of sleep disorders. Washington, DC: American Psychiatric Publishing.

29. Bonnet, M. & Arand, D. (2012). Overview of insomnia: Diagnostic and therapeutic approach. In T.J. Barkoukis, J.K. Matheson, R. Ferber & K. Doghramji (Eds.), Therapy in sleep medicine (pp. 143-150). Philadelphia, PA: Elsevier.

30. Morin, C. M. (2012). Insomnia: prevalence, burden, and consequences. Insomnia Rounds, 1(1), 1-6.

31. Manber, R. & Carney, C. (2015). Treatment plans and interventions for insomnia: A case formulation approach. New York: Guilford Press

32. Chung, F., Yegneswaran, B., Liao, P., Chung, S. A., Vairavanathan, S., Islam, S., ... & Shapiro, C. M. (2008). STOP Questionnaire: A Tool to screen patients for obstructive sleep apnea. Anesthesiology: The Journal of the American Society of Anesthesiologists, 108(5), 812-821.

33. Price, B (2016). Promoting healthy sleep. Nursing Standard, 30(28), 49-58.

34. Macrea, M., Katz, E., Malhotra, A. (2016). Central sleep apnea: Definitions, pathophysiology, genetics, and epidemiology. In M. Kryger, T. Roth & W. Dement (Eds.), Principles and practice of sleep medicine (6th ed., pp. 1049-1075). St. Louis, MO: Elsevier Saunders.

35. Micic, G., Lovato, N., Gradisar, M., Burgess, H. J., Ferguson, S. A., & Lack, L. (2016). Circadian melatonin and temperature taus in delayed sleep-wake phase disorder and non-24-hour sleep-wake rhythm disorder patients: an ultradian constant routine study. Journal of Biological Rhythms, 31(4), 387-405.

36. Wright K., Lowry C., & Lebourgeois M. (2012). Circadian and wakefulness-sleep modulation of cognition in humans. Frontiers in Molecular Neuroscience 5(50), 1-12.

37. Trotti, L. M & Rye, D. B.(2012). Restless legs syndrome and periodic leg movements of sleep. Neurologic Clinics, 30(4), 1137-1166.

38. Mahowald, M. & Bornemann, M. (2011). Non-REM arousal parasomnia. In M. Kryger, T. Roth & W. Dement (Eds.), Principles and practice of sleep medicine (5th ed., pp. 1075-1082). St. Louis, MO: Elsevier.

39. Scammell, T. (2015). Narcolepsy. New England Journal of Medicine, 373(27), 2654-62.

40. Moussavi, S., Chatterji, S., Verdes, E., Tandon, A., Patel, V., & Ustun, B. (2007). Depression, chronic diseases, and decrements in health: Results from the World Health Surveys. The Lancet, 370(9590), 851–858.

41. Taylor, D. J., Lichstein, K. L., Durrence, H. H., Reidel, B. W., & Bush, A. J. (2005). Epidemiology of insomnia, depression, and anxiety. SLEEP 28(11), 1457-1464.

42. Cairns, B. (2007). Alteration of sleep quality by pain medication: An overview. In G. Lavigne, B. J. Sessle, M. Choiniere, & P. J. Soja (Eds.), Sleep and Pain (pp. 371-390). Seattle, WA: IASP Press.

43. Schweitzer, P. & Randazzo, A. (2016). Drugs that disturb sleep and wakefulness. In M. Kryger, T. Roth & W. Dement (Eds.), Principles and practice of sleep medicine (6th ed., pp. 480-498). St. Louis, MO: Elsevier

44. Berterame, S., Erthal, J., Thomas, J., Fellner, S., Vosse, B., Clare, P., ... & Samak, A. K. E. (2016). Use of and barriers to access to opioid analgesics: A worldwide, regional, and national study. The Lancet, 387(10028), 1644-1656.

45. Morasco, B. J., O'hearn, D., Turk, D. C., & Dobscha, S. K. (2014). Associations between prescription opioid use and sleep impairment among veterans with chronic pain. Pain Medicine, 15(11), 1902-1910.

46. Moore, P., Dimsdale J.E. (2002). Opioids, sleep, and cancer-related fatigue. Medical Hypotheses 58(1), 77-82.

47. Van Ryswyk, E., & Antic, N. A. (2016). Opioids and sleep-disordered breathing. Chest, 150(4), 934-944.

48. Schierenbeck, T., Riemann, D., Berger, M., & Hornyak, M. (2008). Effect of illicit recreational drugs upon sleep: Cocaine, ecstasy and marijuana. Sleep Medicine Reviews, 12(5), 381-389.

49. Nicholson, A. N., Turner, C., Stone, B. M., & Robson, P. J. (2004). Effect of Δ-9-Tetrahydrocannabinol and Cannabidiol on nocturnal sleep and early-morning behavior in young adults. Journal of Clinical Psychopharmacology, 24(3), 305-313.

50. Riemann, D., Nissen, C. (2012). Sleep and psychotropic drugs. In C. Morin & C. Espie (Eds.). The Oxford Handbook of Sleep and Sleep Disorders (pp.190-222). New York, NY: Oxford University Press.

51. Sanchez-Ortuno, M., Moore, N., Taillard, J., Valtat, C., Leger, D., Bioulac, B., & Philip, P. (2005). Sleep duration and caffeine consumption in a French middle-aged working population. Sleep Medicine, 6(3), 247–251.

52. Arrigioni, E. & Fuller, P. (2012). An overview of sleep: Physiology and neuroanatomy. In T.J. Barkoukis, J.K. Matheson, R. Ferber & K. Doghramji (Eds.), Therapy in sleep medicine (pp. 43-61). Philadelphia, PA: Elsevier.

53. Roehrs, T. & Roth, T. (2016). Medication and substance abuse. In M. Kryger, T. Roth & W. Dement (Eds.), Principles and practice of sleep medicine (6th ed., pp. 1380-1389). St. Louis, MO: Elsevier

54. Shilo, L., Sabbah, H., Hadari, R., Kovatz, S., & Weinberg, U. (2002). The effects of coffee consumption on sleep and melatonin secretion. Sleep Medicine, 3(3), 271–273.

55. Lavigne, G., Khoury, S., Laverdure-Dupont, D., Denis, R., & Rouleau, G. (2007). Tools and methodological issues in the investigation of sleep and pain interactions. In G. Lavigne, B. J. Sessle, M. Choiniere, & P. J. Soja (Eds.), Sleep and pain (pp. 235-266). Seattle, WA: IASP Press.

56. Haythornthwaite, J. A., Hegel, M. T., & Kerns, R. D. (1991). Development of a sleep diary for chronic pain patients. Journal of Pain and Symptom Management, 6(2), 65-72.

57. Schrimpf, M., Liegl, G., Boeckle, M., Leitner, A., Geisler, P., & Pieh, C. (2015). The effect of sleep deprivation on pain perception in healthy subjects: a meta-analysis. Sleep Medicine, 16(11), 1313-1320.

58. Finan, P. H., Goodin, B. R., & Smith, M. T. (2013). The association of sleep and pain: an update and a path forward. The Journal of Pain, 14(12), 1539-1552.

59. Lautenbacher, S., Kundermann, B. & Krieg, J. (2006). Sleep deprivation and pain perception. Sleep Medicine Reviews, 10, 357–369.

60. Smith, M.T., Perlis, M., Smith, M.S., Giles, D. & Carmody, T. (2000). Sleep quality and presleep arousal in chronic pain. Journal of Behavioral Medicine, 23(1), 1-13.

61. Kundermann, B. & Lautenbacher, S. (2007). Effects of impaired sleep quality and sleep deprivation on diurnal pain perception. In G. Lavigne, B. J. Sessle, M. Choiniere, & P. J. Soja (Eds.), Sleep and pain (pp. 137-152). Seattle, WA: IASP Press.

62. Smith, M. T., & Haythornthwaite, J. A. (2004). How do sleep disturbance and chronic pain inter-relate? Insights from the longitudinal and cognitive-behavioral clinical trials literature. Sleep Medicine Reviews, 8(2), 119-132.

63. Menefee, L. A., Cohen, M. J., Anderson, W. R., Doghramji, K., Frank, E. D., & Lee, H. (2000). Sleep disturbance and nonmalignant chronic pain: a comprehensive review of the literature. Pain Medicine, 1(2), 156-172.

64. Foo, H., & Mason, P. (2003). Brainstem modulation of pain during sleep and waking. Sleep Medicine Reviews, 7(2), 145-154.

65. Shapiro, C., & Girdwood, P. (1981). Protein synthesis in rat brain during sleep. Neuropharmacology, 20(5), 457-460.

66. Culebras, A. (2016). Other neurologic disorders. In M. Kryger, T. Roth & W. Dement (Eds.). Principles and practice of sleep medicine (6th ed., pp. 951-958). St. Louis, MO: Elsevier Saunders.

67. Uhlig, B. L., Engstrøm, M., Ødegård, S. S., Hagen, K. K., & Sand, T. (2014). Headache and insomnia in population-based epidemiological studies. Cephalalgia, 34(10), 745–751.

68. Freedom, T., & Evans, R. W. (2013). Headache and sleep. Headache: The Journal of Head and Face Pain, 53(8), 1358-1366.

69. Ødegård, S. S., Engstrøm, M., Sand, T., Stovner, L. J., Zwart, J. A., & Hagen, K. (2010). Associations between sleep disturbance and primary headaches: The third Nord-Trøndelag Health Study. The Journal of Headache and Pain, 11(3), 197-206

70. Rains, J. & Poceta, S. (2006). Headache and sleep disorders: Review and clinical implications for headache management. Headache: The Journal of Head and Face Pain, 46(9), 12344-1363.

71. Roizenblatt, S., Neto, N. S. R., & Tufik, S. (2011). Sleep disorders and fibromyalgia. Current Pain and Headache Reports, 15(5), 347-357.

72. Castro-Sánchez, A. M., Aguilar-Ferrándiz, M. E., Matarán-Peñarrocha, G. A., del Mar Sánchez-Joya, M., Arroyo-Morales, M., & Fernández-de-las-Peñas, C. (2014). Short-term effects of a manual therapy protocol on pain, physical function, quality of sleep, depressive symptoms, and pressure sensitivity in women and men with fibromyalgia syndrome: a randomized controlled trial. The Clinical Journal of Pain, 30(7), 589-597.

73. Martínez, M. P., Miró, E., Sánchez, A. I., Díaz-Piedra, C., Cáliz, R., Vlaeyen, J. W., & Buela-Casal, G. (2014). Cognitive-behavioral therapy for insomnia and sleep hygiene in fibromyalgia: A randomized controlled trial. Journal of Behavioral Medicine, 37(4), 683-697.

74. Bigatti, S., Hernandez, A., Cronan, T., & Rand, K. (2008). Sleep disturbances in fibromyalgia syndrome: Relationship to pain and depression. Arthritis & Rheumatism, 59(7), 961–967.

75. Nicassio, P. M., & Wallston, K. A. (1992). Longitudinal relationships among pain, sleep problems, and depression in rheumatoid arthritis. Journal of Abnormal Psychology, 101(3), 514-520

76. Hart, F. D., Taylor, R. T., & Huskisson, E. C. (1970). Pain at night. The Lancet, 295(7652), 881-884.

77. Campbell, C. M., Buenaver, L. F., Finan, P., Bounds, S. C., Redding, M., McCauley, L., ... & Smith, M. T. (2015). Sleep, pain catastrophizing, and central sensitization in knee osteoarthritis patients with and without insomnia. Arthritis Care & Research,67(10), 1387-1396.

78. Tishler, M., Barak, Y., Paran, D., & Yaron, M. (1997). Sleep disturbances, fibromyalgia and primary Sjögren's syndrome. Clinical and Experimental Rheumatology, 15(1), 71-74.

79. Wilson, K. G., Eriksson, M. Y., D'Eon, J. L., Mikail, S. F., & Emery, P. C. (2002). Major depression and insomnia in chronic pain. The Clinical Journal of Pain, 18(2), 77–83.

80. Boakye, P. A., Olechowski, C., Rashiq, S., Verrier, M. J., Kerr, B., Witmans, M., ... & Dick, B. D. (2016). A critical review of neurobiological factors involved in the interactions between chronic pain, depression, and sleep disruption. The Clinical Journal of Pain, 32(4), 327-336.

81. Jordan, K. D., & Okifuji, A. (2011). Anxiety disorders: differential diagnosis and their relationship to chronic pain. Journal of Pain & Palliative Care Pharmacotherapy, 25(3), 231–245.

82. Bandelow, B. (2015). Generalized anxiety disorder and pain. In D.P. Finn & B.E. Leonard(Eds.), Pain in psychiatric disorders: Mod trends pharmacopsychiatry (pp 153-165). Basel: Karger AG.

83. Carskadon, M. & Dement, W. (2016). Normal human sleep: An overview. In M. Kryger, T. Roth & W. Dement (Eds.), Principles and practice of sleep medicine (6th ed., pp. 15-24). St. Louis, MO: Elsevier Saunders.

84. Peever, J. H., & McGinty, D. (2007). Why do we sleep? In G. Lavigne, B. J. Sessle, M. Choiniere, & P. J. Soja (Eds.), Sleep and pain (pp. 235-266). Seattle, WA: IASP Press.

85. Siegel, J. (2016). REM Sleep. In M. Kryger, T. Roth & W. Dement (Eds.), Principles and practice of sleep medicine (6th ed., pp. 78-95). St. Louis, MO: Elsevier.

86. Harding, S. (1998). Sleep in fibromyalgia patients: Subjective and objective findings. American Journal of the Medical Sciences 315(6), 367-376.

87. Horne, J. A. (1979). Restitution and human sleep: A critical review. Physiological Psychology, 7(2), 115-125.

88. Berger, M. & Riemann, D. (1993). REM sleep in depression-an overview. Journal of Sleep Research, 2, 211-223.

89. Born J., & Wilhelm, I. (2012). System consolidation of memory during sleep. Psychological Research, 76(2), 192-203

90. Ackermann, S. & Rasch, B. (2014). Differential Effects of Non-REM and REM Sleep on Memory Consolidation? Current Neurology and Neuroscience Reports, 14(2), 430

91. Peigneux, P., Foglel, S., Smith, C. (2016). Memory processing in relation to sleep. In M. Kryger, T. Roth & W. Dement (Eds.), Principles and practice of sleep medicine (6th ed., pp. 229-239). St Louis: Elsevier.

92. Cellini, N. (2017). Memory consolidation in sleep disorders. Sleep Medicine Reviews, 35, 101-112.

93. Rasch, B., & Born, J. (2013). About sleep's role in memory. Physiological Reviews, 93(2), 681-766.

94. Palinkas, L. A., Suefield, P., & Steel, G. D. (1995). Psychological functioning among members of a small polar expedition. Aviation Space and Environmental Medicine, 66, 943-950.

95. Orr, W. C., Altshuler, K.Z., & Stahl, M.L. (1982). Managing sleep complaints. Chicago, IL: Year Book Medical Publishers.

96. Horne, J. (2011). The end of sleep: 'Sleep debt' versus biological adaptation of human sleep to waking needs. Biological Psychology, 87(1), 1-14

97. Bliwise, D. (2011). Normal aging. In M. Kryger, T. Roth & W. Dement (Eds.), Principles and practice of sleep medicine (5th ed., pp. 27-41). St. Louis, MO: Elsevier Saunders.

98. Borbely, A., Daan, S., Wirz-Justice, A. & Deboer, T. (2016). The two-process model of sleep regulation: A reappraisal. Journal of Sleep Research, 25(2), 131-143.

99. Richardson, G. S. (2005). The human circadian system in normal and disordered sleep. The Journal of Clinical Psychiatry, 66(suppl. 9), 3-9.

100. Hastings, M., O'Neill, J. S., & Maywood, E. S. (2007). Circadian clocks: regulators of endocrine and metabolic rhythms. Journal of Endocrinology, 195(2), 187-198.

101. Dijk, D. J., & Lockley, S. W. (2002). Invited Review: Integration of human sleep-wake regulation and circadian rhythmicity. Journal of Applied Physiology, 92(2), 852-862.

102. Regestein, Q., Natarajan, V., Pavlova, M., Kawasaki, S., Gleason, R., & Koff, E. (2010). Sleep debt and depression in female college students. Psychiatry Research, 176(1), 34-39.

103. Horne, J., Anderson, C., & Platten, C. (2008). Sleep extension versus nap or coffee, within the context of 'sleep debt'. Journal of Sleep Research, 17(4), 432-436.

104. Mollayeva, T., Thurairajah, P., Burton, K., Mollayeva, S., Shapiro, C., & Colantonio, A. (2016). The Pittsburgh sleep quality index as a screening tool for sleep dysfunction in clinical and non-clinical samples: A systematic review and meta-analysis. Sleep Medicine Review, 25, 52-73.

105. Buysse, D. J., Reynolds, C. F., Monk, T. H., Berman, S. R., & Kupfer, D. J. (1989). The Pittsburgh sleep quality index: A new instrument for psychiatric practice and research. Psychiatry Research, 28(2), 193-213.

106. Cole, J. C., Dubois, D., & Kosinski, M. (2007). Use of patient-reported sleep measures in clinical trials of pain treatment: A literature review and synthesis of current sleep measures and a conceptual model of sleep disturbance in pain. Clinical Therapy, 29, 2580-2588.

107. Johns, M. W. (1991). A new method for measuring daytime sleepiness: The Epworth sleepiness scale. SLEEP, 14(6), 540-545

108. Smith, M. T., & Wegener, S. T. (2003). Measures of sleep: the insomnia severity index, medical outcomes study (MOS) sleep scale, Pittsburgh sleep diary (PSD), and Pittsburgh sleep quality index (PSQI). Arthritis & Rheumatology 49(S5), S184 - S196

109. Morin, C.M. (1993). Insomnia: psychological assessment and management. New York, NY: Guilford Press

110. Carney, C., Buysse, D., Ancoli-Israel, S., Edinger, J., Krystal, A., et al (2012). The consensus sleep diary: Standardizing prospective sleep self-monitoring. SLEEP, 35(2), 287-302.

111. Edinger, J., Means, M., Carney, C. & Manber, R. (2011). Psychological and behavioral treatments for insomnia II: Implementation and specific populations. In M. Kryger, T. Roth & W. Dement (Eds.), Principles and practice of sleep medicine (5th ed., pp. 884-904). St Louis: Elsevier.

112. Morin, C. M., Vallieres, A., & Ivers, H. (2007). Dysfunctional beliefs and attitudes about sleep (DBAS), Validation of a brief version (DBAS-16). SLEEP, 30(11), 1547-1554.

113. Carskadon, M. A., Dement, W. C., Mitler, M. M., Roth, T., Westbrook, P. R., & Keenan, S. (1986). Guidelines for the Multiple Sleep Latency Test (MSLT): A standard measure of sleepiness. Sleep, 9(4), 519-524.

114. Sadeh, A. (2011). The role and validity of actigraphy in sleep medicine: An update. Sleep Medicine Reviews, 15(4), 259–267.

115. Haggmann, S., Maher, C. & Refshauge, K. (2004). Screening for symptoms of depression by physical therapists managing low back pain. Physical Therapy, 84(12), 1-10.

116. Masters, P. A. (2014). Insomnia. Annals of Internal Medicine, 161(7), ITC1-ITC15.

117. Flemons, W. W., Douglas, N. J., Kuna, S. T., Rodenstein, D. O., & Wheatley, J. (2004). Access to diagnosis and treatment of patients with suspected sleep apnea. American Journal of Respiratory and Critical Care Medicine, 169(6), 668-672.

118. Schutte-Rodin, S., Broch, L., Buysse, D., Dorsey, C., & Sateia, M. (2008). Clinical guideline for the evaluation and management of chronic insomnia in adults. Journal of Clinical Sleep Medicine 4(5), 487-504.

119. Greenberg, H., Lakticova, V. & Scharf., S. (2016). Obstructive sleep apnea: Clinical features, evaluation, and principles of management. In M. Kryger, T.

Roth & W. Dement (Ed.), Principles and practice of sleep medicine (6th ed., pp. 432-445). St Louis: Elsevier.

120. Walsh, J., Roth, T. (2016). Pharmacologic treatment of insomnia: Benzodiazepine receptor agonists. In M. Kryger, T. Roth & W. Dement (Eds.), Principles and practice of sleep medicine (6th ed., pp. 832-841). St Louis: Elsevier

121. Trauer, J. M., Qian, M. Y., Doyle, J. S., Rajaratnam, S. M., & Cunnington, D. (2015). Cognitive behavioral therapy for chronic insomnia: A systematic review and meta-analysis. Annals of Internal Medicine, 163(3), 191-204.

122. DynaMed Plus [Internet]. Ipswich (MA): EBSCO Information Services. 1995 - . Record No. 905574, Choosing Wisely Canada; [updated 2016 Oct 26, cited Edmonton, AB September 21, 2017]; Available from http://www.dynamed.com/login.aspx?direct=true&site=DynaMed&id=905574. Registration and login required.

123. Mitchell, M. D., Gehrman, P., Perlis, M., & Umscheid, C. A. (2012). Comparative effectiveness of cognitive behavioral therapy for insomnia: a systematic review. BMC Family Practice, 13(1), 40-50

124. Nalajala, N., Walls, K., & Hili, E. (2013). Insomnia in chronic lower back pain: Non-pharmacological physiotherapy interventions. International Journal of Therapy and Rehabilitation, 20(10), 510-516.

125. Hauri, P. (2012). Sleep/wake lifestyle modifications: Sleep hygiene. In T.J. Barkoukis, J.K. Matheson, R. Ferber & K. Doghramji (Eds.), Therapy in sleep medicine (pp. 151-160). Philadelphia, PA: Elsevier.

126. Hoch, C. C., Reynolds III, C. F., Buysse, D. J., Monk, T. H., Nowell, P., Begley, A. E., ... & Dew, M. A. (2001). Protecting sleep quality in later life: A pilot study of bed restriction and sleep hygiene. The Journals of Gerontology Series B: Psychological Sciences and Social Sciences, 56(1), 52-59.

127. Morin, C., Davidson, J. & Beaulieu-Bonneau, S. (2016). Cognitive behavior therapies for insomnia I: Approaches and efficacy. In M. Kryger, T. Roth & W. Dement (Eds.), Principles and practice of sleep medicine (6th ed., pp. 804-813). St Louis: Elsevier

128. Stepanski, E. & Wyatt, J. (2003). Use of sleep hygiene in the treatment of insomnia. Sleep Medicine Reviews, 7(3),215-225

129. Jacobs, G., Pace-Schott, E., Stickgold, R., & Otto, M. (2004). Cognitive behavior therapy and pharmacotherapy for insomnia: A randomized controlled trial and direct comparison. Archives of Internal Medicine, 164(17), 1888-1896.

130. Irish, L. A., Kline, C. E., Gunn, H. E., Buysse, D. J., & Hall, M. H. (2015). The role of sleep hygiene in promoting public health: A review of empirical evidence. Sleep Medicine Reviews, 22, 23–36.

131. Christensen, M. A., Bettencourt, L., Kaye, L., Moturu, S. T., Nguyen, K. T., Olgin, J. E., ... & Marcus, G. M. (2016). Direct measurements of smartphone screen-time: relationships with demographics and sleep. PLoS One, 11(11), e0165331. doi: 10.1371/journal.pone.0165331

132. Dzierzewski, J. M., Buman, M. P., Giacobbi, P. R., Roberts, B. L.,-Aiken-Morgan, A. T., Marsiske, M., & McCrae, C. S. (2014). Exercise and sleep in community-dwelling older adults: evidence for a reciprocal relationship. Journal of Sleep Research, 23(1), 61-68.

133. Lambiase, M., Gabriel, K., Kuller, L. & Matthews, K. (2013). Temporal relationships between physical activity and sleep in older women. Medicine and Science in Sports and Exercise, 45(12), 1-14.

134. Yang, P. Y., Ho, K. H., Chen, H. C., & Chien, M. Y. (2012). Exercise training improves sleep quality in middle-aged and older adults with sleep problems: A systematic review. Journal of Physiotherapy, 58(3), 157-163.

135. Reid, K., Baron, K., Lu, B., Naylor, E., Wolfe, L. & Zee, P. (2010). Aerobic exercise improves self-reported sleep and quality of life in older adults with insomnia. Sleep Medicine, 11(9), 934-940.

136. Madden, K. M., Ashe, M. C., Lockhart, C., & Chase, J. M. (2014). Sedentary behavior and sleep efficiency in active community-dwelling older adults. Sleep Science, 7(2), 82-88.

137. Oudegeest-Sander, M. H., Eijsvogels, T. H., Verheggen, R. J., Poelkens, F., Hopman, M. T., Jones, H., & Thijssen, D. H. (2013). Impact of physical fitness and daily energy expenditure on sleep efficiency in young and older humans. Gerontology, 59(1), 8-16.

138. de Castro Toledo Guimaraes, L., de Carvalho L.B., Yanaguibashi G. & do Prado, G. (2008). Physically active elderly women sleep more and better than sedentary women. Sleep Medicine, 9(5),488-93.

139. Giebelhaus, V., Strohl, K. P., Lormes, W., Lehmann, M., & Netzer, N. (2000). Physical exercise as an adjunct therapy in sleep apnea—an open trial. Sleep and Breathing, 4(4), 173-176.

140. Neuendorf, R., Wahbeh, H., Chamine, I., Yu, J., Hutchison, K., & Oken, B. S. (2015). The effects of mind-body interventions on sleep quality: A systematic

review. Evidence-Based Complementary and Alternative Medicine, 2015(2), 1–17.

141. Sarris, J., & Byrne, G. J. (2011). A systematic review of insomnia and complementary medicine. Sleep Medicine Reviews, 15(2), 99–106.

142. Bertisch, S. M., Wells, R. E., Smith, M. T., & McCarthy, E. P. (2017). Use of relaxation techniques and complementary and alternative medicine by American adults with insomnia symptoms: Results from a national survey. Journal of Clinical Sleep Medicine, 8(6), 681–691.

143. Martires, J., & Zeidler, M. (2015). The value of mindfulness meditation in the treatment of insomnia. Current Opinion in Pulmonary Medicine, 21(6), 547–552.

144. Black D, O'Reilly G, Olmstead R, Breen E, Irwin M (2015). Mindfulness meditation and improvement in sleep quality and daytime impairment among older adults with sleep disturbances: a randomized clinical trial. JAMA Internal Medicine, 175(4), 494 – 501

145. Ong, J. C., Manber, R., Segal, Z., Xia, Y., Shapiro, S., & Wyatt, J. K. (2014). A randomized controlled trial of mindfulness meditation for chronic insomnia. SLEEP, 37(9), 1553-1563.

146. Boettcher, J., Åström, V., Påhlsson, D., Schenström, O., Andersson, G., & Carlbring, P. (2014). Internet-based mindfulness treatment for anxiety disorders: A randomized controlled trial. Behavior Therapy, 45(2), 241-253.

147. Garland, S. N., Carlson, L. E., Stephens, A. J., Antle, M. C., Samuels, C., & Campbell, T. S. (2014). Mindfulness-based stress reduction compared with cognitive behavioral therapy for the treatment of insomnia comorbid with cancer: a randomized, partially blinded, noninferiority trial. Journal of Clinical Oncology, 32(5), 449-457.

148. Irwin, M., Olmstead, R., & Motivala, S. (2008). Improving sleep in older adults with moderate sleep complaints: A randomized controlled trial of Tai Chi. SLEEP 31(7), 1001-1008.

149. Rose, K., Bourguignon, C. (2011). Complementary and alternative medicine and sleep. In N. Redeker & G. McEnany (Eds.) Sleep disorders and sleep promotion in nursing practice (pp 233-242). New York, NY: Springer Publishing.

150. Manjunath, N. K., & Telles, S. (2005). Influence of Yoga & Ayurveda on self-rated sleep in a geriatric population. Indian Journal of Medical Research, 121(5), 683-690

151. Shergis, J. L., Ni, X., Jackson, M. L., Zhang, A. L., Guo, X., Li, Y., ... & Xue, C. C. (2016). A systematic review of acupuncture for sleep quality in people with insomnia. Complementary Therapies in Medicine, 26, 11-20.

152. Juarascio, A., Cuellar, N. & Gooneratne, N. (2012). Alternative therapeutics for sleep disorders. In T.J. Barkoukis, J.K. Matheson, R. Ferber & K. Doghramji (Eds.), Therapy in sleep medicine (pp. 126-137). Philadelphia, PA: Elsevier.

153. Krystal, A. (2016). Pharmacologic treatment of insomnia: Other medications. In M. Kryger, T. Roth & W. Dement (Eds.), Principles and practice of sleep medicine (6th ed., pp 842-854). St Louis: Elsevier.

154. Buysse, D. & Tyagi, S. (2016). Clinical pharmacology of other drugs used as hypnotics. In M. Kryger, T. Roth & W. Dement (Eds.), Principles and practice of sleep medicine (6th ed., pp. 432-445). St Louis: Elsevier.

155. Morin, C., Bootzin, R., Buysse, D., Edinger, J., Espie, C. & Lichstein K. (2006). Psychological and behavioral treatment of insomnia: Update of the recent evidence (1998-2004). SLEEP, 29(11), 1398-1414.

156. Manber, R., Carney, C., Edinger, J., Epstein, D., Friedman, L., Haynes, P. L., et al. (2012). Dissemination of CBTI to the Non-Sleep Specialist: Protocol Development and Training Issues. Journal of Clinical Sleep Medicine, 8(2): 209-218.

157. Espie, C. (2009). "Stepped care": A health technology solution for delivering cognitive behavorial therapy as a first line insomnia treatment. SLEEP, 32(12), 1549-1558.

158. Seyffert, M., Lagisetty, P., Landgraf, J., Chopra, V., Pfeiffer, P. N., Conte, M. L., & Rogers, M. A. (2016). Internet-delivered cognitive behavioral therapy to treat insomnia: A systematic review and meta-analysis. PLoS One, 11(2), e0149139. doi:10.1371/journal.pone.0149139

159. Espie, C. & Kyle, S. (2012). Cognitive behavioral and psychological therapies for chronic insomnia. In T.J. Barkoukis, J.K. Matheson, R. Ferber & K. Doghramji (Eds.), Therapy in sleep medicine (pp. 161-171). Philadelphia, PA: Elsevier

160. Riemann, D., Spiegelhalder, K., Feige, B., Voderholzer, U., Berger, M., Perlis, M., & Nissen, C. (2010). The hyperarousal model of insomnia: a review of the concept and its evidence. Sleep Medicine Reviews, 14(1), 19-31.

161. Harvey, A. (2002). A cognitive model of insomnia. Behavior Research and Therapy, 40, 869-893

www.ingramcontent.com/pod-product-compliance
Lightning Source LLC
Chambersburg PA
CBHW052133270326
41930CB00012B/2862